COPING WITH A HERNIA

DR DAVID DELVIN is director of the Medical Information Service, and one of Britain's best-known media doctors. He trained in medicine at King's College Hospital, London, and subsequently worked at hospitals in Sussex, Kent and West Indies. After becoming a member of the Royal College of General Practitioners, he established a successful career in writing and broadcasting about medicine and surgery. He has now appeared in over 800 medical TV programmes. His work has received awards from the Medical Journalists' Association and the American Medical Writers' Association. He has also been Consumer Columnist of the Year, and he was awarded the *Médaille de la Ville de Paris* by Jacques Chirac.

Overcoming Common Problems Series

For a full list of titles please contact
Sheldon Press, Marylebone Road, London NW1 4DU

Overcoming Common Problems Series

Overcoming Common Problems Series

Overcoming Common Problems

Coping with a Hernia

Dr David Delvin

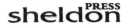

sheldon **PRESS**

First published in Great Britain in 1998 by Sheldon Press,
SPCK, Holy Trinity Church, Marylebone Road, London NW1 4DU

© David Delvin 1998

British Library Cataloguing-in-Publication Data
A catalogue for this book is available from the British Library

ISBN 0–85969–783–5

Photoset by Deltatype Limited, Birkenhead, Merseyside
Printed in Great Britain by
Biddles Ltd, Guildford and King's Lynn

Contents

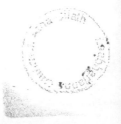

Acknowledgements

My grateful thanks to the following people and organizations who have helped me with information for this book:

Press Department, Royal College of Surgeons of England
Matthew Nolan, Orthotist, Surgical Appliance Department, Addenbrooke's Hospital
Mr David Dunn, M Chir, FRCS
Mr Mitchell Notaras, FRCS, FRCS Ed, FACS
Leslie Seldon, Solicitor, Messrs Clarkson, Wright & Jakes
Peter Boyes, Niche Communications Ltd

Introduction

The unfortunate thing about having a hernia is that in general people don't take this condition very seriously.

So unless you're lucky, you may not get much sympathy from your family or friends – or indeed your boss.

Sadly, the condition has become something of a music-hall joke in many people's minds. I once told a man that his wife had a pretty bad hernia, and instead of being sympathetic he replied, 'She should never have gone to that Ivor Novello musical; you know, doc: *Careless Rupture.*' His wife was not amused.

On another occasion, I informed a father that his young son was suffering from a groin hernia. He embarrassed the boy by laughing heartily and saying, 'Don't worry, old chap – we belong to the National Truss.'

But the truth is that hernias (ruptures) can be distressing, debilitating and painful – so they're no laughing matter. Very occasionally they even cost patients their lives, sometimes as a result of the warning symptoms being neglected – either by patient or doctor.

It's silly that this common condition isn't taken more seriously, and it's crazy that there's so much *embarrassment* about it. Because of this embarrassment, some men and women hide their hernias away for months or years – not going to a doctor till they're in desperate trouble. That is not wise . . .

Looking on the bright side, the last few years have brought enormous advances in hernia treatment – advances which have helped many people get out of hospital a lot faster, with a lot less pain and disability. You can find out about these advances from this book.

Also, in the last year or two it has become much commoner for patients to play a part in *choosing* what sort of hernia treatment they have.

If you want to be a partner (with your GP or surgeon) in making that sort of choice, rather than just accepting that 'the doctors know best', then read on.

Note: 'he' and 'she', referring to patients or doctors, have been used randomly and thus (I hope) inclusively throughout the book (except where a condition applies only to one sex – and in the case of hernia surgeons who remain almost exclusively male).

1

What is a hernia – and what can be done about it?

The first thing to say about a hernia is that the word means exactly the same thing as a 'rupture'. A lot of people think that the two expressions refer to different disorders, but they don't. Hernia is just the Latin word for rupture.

But what actually *is* a hernia? I find that many patients are extremely confused about this. That's not surprising, because accurate information about ruptures is quite hard to obtain.

For instance, one dictionary's definition begins with the chilling words, 'A tumour, usually in the groin'. This is wildly misleading, because most people interpret the word tumour as meaning a cancer. In fact, its true meaning is a swelling or lump – and that's exactly what a hernia is.

A hernia is actually a swelling caused by part of you bulging out through a gap. Hernias can occur in all sorts of places in the body, but in every case what happens is the same: there's a weakness somewhere, and one of your organs bulges through it, causing a swelling.

You can get a good idea of what a hernia is by taking a toy balloon and blowing it up till it's about the size of an orange. Then hold it between your two hands, with your fingers interlaced, so that the balloon is more or less hidden. Now squeeze your hands together gently, so that you put pressure on it; then allow a little gap to appear between your fingers. The balloon will immediately start bulging through the gap. This is exactly what happens with a hernia: something which is under pressure manages to force its way through a tiny gap.

In real life, it's often a bit of intestine which is trying to push its way through a gap. (Incidentally, the word 'intestine' means exactly the same thing as 'gut' or 'bowel' – it's the tubing through which your digested food passes.)

Hernias can occur in all sorts of different places, as you can see from Figure 1. Wherever there is a small aperture in the body, it's possible for some structure to try and force its way through the gap. So you can have a hernia coming through your navel, causing a bulge under your skin – or through the weakened scar of a surgical operation (this is called an incisional hernia). All of these non-groin ruptures are dealt with fully in Chapter 11. However, this book does *not* deal with a very different sort of condition called hiatus hernia – this is covered by a companion volume in the Overcoming Common Problems series (*Coping Successfully with a Hiatus Hernia*).

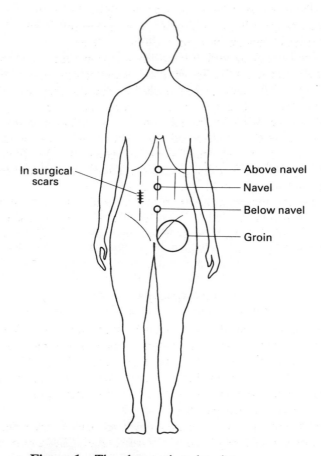

In surgical scars

Above navel

Navel

Below navel

Groin

Figure 1   The places where hernias occur.

A bulge in the groin

Well over 85 per cent of hernias occur in the groin region – so the next few chapters will be about ruptures in that particular area. However, since I find that people are sometimes a trifle uncertain as to what the word 'groin' actually means, let me make it quite clear. It doesn't mean the sex organs (a common misunderstanding). The groin is actually the zone just to one side of the sexual parts – right where the abdomen (belly) meets the thigh.

Now the human body is curiously weak in that region – for reasons which we'll go into shortly. That's why it's extraordinarily easy for the intestine to shove its way through a defect in the groin and cause a bulge. It's so easy, in fact, that at least one in eight of us will get a groin rupture at some time in our lives.

Although hernias are very common, many people are embarrassed about having them. I have known patients pretend to their families that they are having an appendix operation, because they don't like to mention the word rupture. Such embarrassment seems to stem mainly from the fact that groin hernias occur so close to the sex organs. Also, there's a widespread myth that ruptures are connected with sex: they're not – except in some very minor details which are explained in Chapter 9. Having a hernia doesn't mean that you're likely to start having trouble with your love-life.

So please try and put any embarrassment aside. If you think you may have a hernia, don't hide it away. There's nothing shameful about it – so don't hesitate to go along to your doctor and have it checked out. The sooner it's treated, the better!

Treatment

How are hernias treated? Unfortunately there are no tablets or medicines to make everything better. People sometimes ask if alternative medication would help, but that really isn't possible. This is one small area of medical practice where complementary treatment can do nothing – though a few alternative practitioners claim otherwise (see Chapter 8).

The treatment of ruptures comes down to one of three things: having an operation, being fitted with a truss, or adopting a wait-and-see policy.

5

1 Having an operation

The purpose of the operation is to mend the defect in your groin, so that you no longer have a swelling there. Most people who have hernias are treated in this way. But (as we'll see in a moment) there are now various types of operation – and it's worth your while to know about them and, where possible, to exercise your choice.

2 Being fitted with a truss

A truss is a groin support, rather like a low-slung belt. The idea is that the pressure of the truss keeps the hernia more or less under control – in other words, stops it from bulging out. Trusses do not cure hernias, but they can help ease discomfort.

However, you'll find that doctors in general tend to be rather against the idea of their patients using a truss. This is mainly because they know that serious complications quite often occur in hernias which haven't been surgically repaired. In addition, there are some groin hernias which simply cannot be controlled by a truss. There is more about trusses in Chapter 8 – do not spend your money on one till you have read that chapter!

3 Adopting a wait-and-see policy

It's sometimes possible just to keep a small hernia under medical observation – in other words, to do nothing for the time being. The main reason for taking this approach would be if the person is so old and infirm that it would be distressing or dangerous for him to undergo surgery. For instance, in England the Royal College of Surgeons has recently issued guidelines which say that *small* groin ruptures of one particular type do not always have to be operated on, especially if the patient is elderly.

However, surgeons in some parts of the world take the view that all groin hernias should be surgically repaired, if at all possible – because of the risk that problems may arise.

Warning note: If you decide not to have an operation on your hernia, it is important that you should have it checked from time to time by a doctor. And it is *vital* that you seek urgent medical advice if you develop pain in the region of the rupture, or if you start vomiting for no obvious reason.

Recent improvements in surgery

Recently, things have been changing very fast in the field of hernia treatment. One of the biggest changes has been that patients are now starting to make choices for themselves. They're beginning to decide which surgeon will treat them, and which type of operation they will have.

Until just a few years ago, must rupture patients had virtually no choice about their treatment. What happened if you had a hernia was this:

- You went to your GP;
- She confirmed the diagnosis, and wrote a letter for you to take to the surgeon at the nearest hospital;
- After some weeks or months, the surgeon saw you, examined you – and then put you on the end of a long waiting list;
- When you eventually got to the top of that waiting list, the surgeon got you into hospital, where he carried out a traditional hernia repair operation. This is rather like darning a hole in an old sock, and is a procedure which has remained virtually unchanged for many years. There's a certain amount of pain afterwards, and recovery from the operation is quite slow. For instance, back in the 1970s, some surgeons kept patients in hospital for as much as 12 days post-operatively – though by the 1990s hospital stays had become much shorter.

As you can see, most patients had very little choice in this process: you got the surgeon to whom your GP sent you, you had the 'traditional' operation – and that was that.

But in the last few years, the following new factors have come into play.

1 The need for patients to get out of hospital faster. Surgeons and hospitals now want to get you in and out as fast as possible. This is less for the benefit of the patient, and more for financial considerations. However, many patients are delighted to be discharged from hospital soon after their operations (though some aren't – see Chapter 12).

The speeding-up process has encouraged surgeons to start using newer operations which have a quicker recovery time. It has also

7

encouraged both GPs and patients to shop around for hospitals which have a quicker through-put of patients.

2 The development of keyhole surgery. Keyhole or laparoscopic surgery – which is fully explained in Chapter 5 – has been used fairly successfully in many fields for a long time now. But in recent years, it has been applied to hernia treatment.

During a keyhole operation, the surgeon works through very tiny incisions. So the patient's recovery time is usually very quick – mainly because there is no long, painful cut to heal up.

3 The development of the 'mesh technique' (also called the open mesh operation). Some surgeons have recently claimed excellent results for a revolutionary surgical method. Instead of darning up the gap through which the rupture passes, they insert a small sheet of synthetic mesh, rather smaller than a playing card in size. Full details are given in Chapter 5. The operation can easily be done under local anaesthetic, which makes it popular with patients – as does the fact that you can normally go home the same day.

4 The wider use of private medicine. Whether or not you approve of this, the fact is that a lot more people have opted for private hernia surgery in Britain in recent years. One cause of this trend has been the great length of many hospital waiting lists. If you are going to suffer discomfort for many months before you can get a hernia operation on the National Health Service (NHS), it's very tempting to go to a private clinic, if you can afford it. Currently, most private hernia clinics are using the new mesh technique, but this may change as other operations come in (see Chapter 5).

Note: If you go to a private hospital, be sure it's a safe, well-equipped and reputable one. Be guided by your GP. Most importantly, could the hospital cope if anything went wrong during your surgery?

5 The establishment of specialist hernia centres. Until recently, all rupture operations were done by surgeons whose field is *general* surgery. So your hernia operation might have been done at the end of a busy operating session which had included (say) a gall-bladder removal, a bowel cancer operation, and a couple of cases of piles. Very often, the consultant surgeon actually departed, and your operation was done by one of the junior doctors. So no matter how talented the surgeon – or the junior – might be, you were not being treated by a hernia specialist.

The advent of private hernia centres has changed a lot of people's views of this operation. Suddenly, it seems fashionable to be operated on by a surgeon whose main interest is ruptures, and who does little else but this type of surgery. In 1997, the first NHS unit exclusively for treating hernias opened in Plymouth, and others were to follow.

Will a large number of NHS hernia units open? That depends very much on whether they turn out to save money! At present, there are some indications that they will, simply because a specialist hernia service gets patients in and out quickly. Also, it is claimed that a rupture which is repaired by a hernia specialist (as opposed to a general surgeon) is less likely to recur.

Sadly, many hernias do recur some years after an operation. If the new centres really do have lower recurrence rates, then that will clearly be an economic saving – so the specialized units will flourish.

However, for the time being most hernia sufferers in Britain and Ireland are seen by a general surgeon – and in most cases, the operation is done perfectly competently.

However, there is a very strong case for asking your GP to send you to the surgeon who has the best local reputation for hernia repairs. And you should most definitely enquire whether the surgeon is using one of the newer techniques mentioned in this book.

And if you're feeling brave, you should also ask how much experience the surgeon has in using the new technique. To go to someone who only started doing it last week is probably not a very bright idea.

2

Groin hernias – the causes

In the UK, about 80,000 people a year have surgery for groin hernias. Why are ruptures in this area of the body so common? What causes them?

Let's look first of all at why people *think* they happen. While preparing this book, I did a small survey among patients, in which I asked them what they thought had caused their hernias. Their replies included:

- 'It just happens';
- 'Exercise';
- 'Sitting in a funny way at work';
- 'Tough manual labour';
- 'Probably sex';
- 'Gardening, I suppose';
- 'Eating the wrong sort of food';
- 'Lifting a parcel for my boss';
- 'All that commuting to work'.

Most of the above answers are wrong – though the people who mentioned lifting and heavy work were beginning to get on the right track (we'll look at the role of lifting and physical effort later in this chapter). But the main reason why so many groin ruptures occur is that our bodies are potentially rather weak in that particular area – and that's especially true of the male human body. Furthermore, most surgeons believe that the majority of hernias develop because the person was born with an excessively weak groin region. In other words, many hernias are congenital – even though lifting and heavy work may make the bulge actually appear.

The groin's natural weakness

The human groin is an area of potential weakness for two anatomical reasons:

- Because it's a 'joining' region of the body;

- Because there have to be holes in it (though you can't actually see these yourself – they're under the skin).

Any join in the body is a place where things can go wrong. Your groin is the zone where your abdomen (belly) meets your thigh. And – just like a join in a roof or wall – it's therefore a place where things tend to come apart.

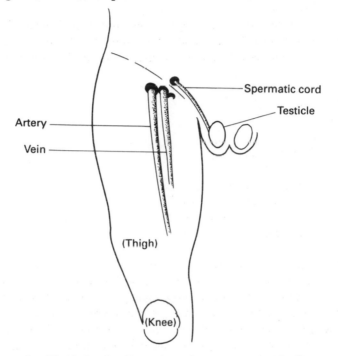

Figure 2 The holes in the groin – these are anatomically essential, but increase the risk of a hernia.

Furthermore, the groin is pierced by several holes. They have to be there because, as you can see from Figure 2, there are several important blood-carrying tubes (arteries and veins) which, together with other structures like nerves, leave your abdomen in the groin area and run down into your leg. There is also a hole in the groin through which the spermatic cord passes – as you'll see from Figure 2, this is the 'plumbing' that runs down to the testicle. Women also have that particular hole, but it is smaller – and that simple fact explains why ruptures are much commoner in men than they are in women.

So all of us have gaps in the groin through which a hernia could push itself. But in addition to this, large numbers of people are actually born with an extra weakness, as shown in Figure 3. It's a little pouch or sac of tissue which projects through one of the holes – rather as if a tiny finger-stall or condom were poking through it. This bag-like projection is practically inviting your intestine to slip into it.

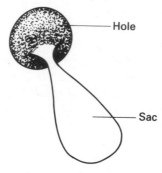

Figure 3   The congenital sac or pouch, which increases the risk of a hernia.

If you have this congenital pouch in your groin, then it is very likely that at some time in your life you will get a hernia. Whether you do so or not will depend on various factors.

Note: A 'double' hernia is not a very common condition. It simply means that you have two hernias – one on each side.

Other factors

There are various other factors which tend to provoke hernias – especially in people who have the congenital sac, but also in the rest of us. Let's look at them one by one.

1 Lifting

People who think that hernias are something to do with lifting are right – at least, in many cases.

The reason is that when you lift a heavy weight the pressure inside your abdomen increases greatly. Remember the demonstration with the toy balloon (in Chapter 1): when you increased the pressure on the balloon, it was much more likely to bulge out between your fingers. In exactly the same way, lifting creates such a lot of pressure that it tends to shove your intestines out through any weak spot. As we've seen, the groin is just such an area – especially if you have a congenital sac.

But can one single, heavy lift provoke a rupture, as people often think? This is very hard to say. Sometimes a person lifts a massive weight and feels something 'go' in the groin; afterwards a rupture is diagnosed – but was it there beforehand or did it occur at the time of the lift? It's almost impossible to prove either way.

Similarly, it is very common for people whose jobs involve repeated lifting to claim that their ruptures are due to their occupation. Understandably, they may well try to sue their employers. However, in practice it is quite difficult to succeed with this type of legal action, because of the problem of *proving* that repeated lifting actually causes the hernia. The employers' lawyers will almost certainly obtain an expert opinion from a consultant surgeon who will say that the main problem was a pre-existing weakness in the person's groin. However, suing a *negligent* employer (for example, one who has asked you to lift unreasonably heavy weights without assistance) is far from impossible; Clarkson, Wright & Jakes, a noted firm of medico-legal solicitors, tell me that awards in recent years have varied between £1,500 and – most exceptionally – £90,000.

It's even more difficult to claim that a hernia was due to general heavy work (without a lot of lifting). Although almost any kind of straining increases abdominal pressure, it would be very hard to prove that this was the cause of the rupture. None the less, a number of people have successfully claimed that non-lifting strains were the cause of their hernias, and have been awarded damages.

2 Being overweight

There's no doubt that being fat increases your chances of developing a hernia, especially if the weakness is already there.

Whether being just a few pounds overweight makes much difference is uncertain. Many doctors would say that staying slim is a good way of reducing your chances of a hernia – though it's not a foolproof method, as many thin people also get them.

It is certain, though, that the more obese you are, the more difficult your hernia operation is likely to be.

3 Poor abdominal muscles

If you let your tummy muscles get out of shape, this increases the chances of having a hernia. Sadly, many people's abdominal muscles do get flabby and lax over the years, particularly as a result of:

- childbirth;
- inactivity;
- being overweight.

If you have developed a bit of a paunch in recent years, then it's more than likely that the muscles of your lower belly are in poor condition. Building them up – for instance, by working out at a gym, or even just doing daily sit-ups at home – may possibly reduce your chances of developing a rupture. But exercises can't cure a rupture, once it has occurred.

4 Repeated coughing

If you have chest trouble and keep coughing repeatedly over a long period of time, that too can increase your chances of getting a rupture. We're not talking here about the kind of winter cough that's over in a week or so – *that* won't give you a hernia. But if you have (say) chronic bronchitis and keep coughing endlessly for months or years, then that causes repeated surges in your abdominal pressure, and the eventual result may be that your poor, battered groin gives way under the strain.

Obviously, any long-term cough needs investigation and treatment. If a cough goes on for more than a week or so, you should always see your doctor.

5 'Straining at stool'

The medical term 'straining at stool' means straining while you're trying to open your bowels. Quite a lot of people do deliberately push downwards very hard when sitting on the loo. They're specially likely to do this if they're constipated.

That kind of straining produces a phenomenal rise in abdominal pressure. So if you have a weakness in the groin, this type of repeated straining may well make it into a rupture. The moral is: do not strain at stool. And avoid constipation by eating a lot of fruit, vegetables, cereals and wholemeal bread.

6 Straining to pass urine

This particular hernia-provoking factor is only relevant to older men who have prostate trouble – but there are an awful lot of them!

If you keep forcing downwards in order to try and pass water, that pumps up the pressure inside your abdomen – and, as we've seen, a rise in pressure may easily push a bulge out through any weakness you may have in your groin.

If you have difficulty in peeing, please see a doctor for investigation and treatment.

Summary

In summary, the factors which may provoke a hernia in someone who has a weakness in the groin are: lifting, obesity, weak abdominal muscles, repeated coughing, and straining to pass bowel motions or urine.

I've occasionally known people blame other things for their ruptures – such as stress, a powerful orgasm, golf, being unable to pass wind for social reasons, or lack of vitamins. None of these can cause a hernia. For completeness, I should add that I once saw a patient who claimed that he had been 'ruptured' by a surgeon who did a rectal examination on him. That too is impossible.

3

Discovering a groin hernia – and what to do about it

So how do you know if you've got a groin hernia? What are the symptoms?

There are several possible symptoms, but much the commonest is a lump located in your groin – in other words, a few centimetres to the right or left of the sex organs.

Finding a lump

You may first notice a lump when you're washing or having a bath. You might accidentally feel it with your finger-tips, or you might just look down one day and see that there's a slight bulge round about the edge of the triangle of pubic hair. Some people's reaction is to panic – but there's no need for this. After all, if it's a hernia it will almost certainly be curable. But it is very important that you go to your doctor within the next few days and have the lump checked out.

Most uncommonly, the lump is very painful – and in that case, you should contact your GP immediately – because you need to be examined within the next few hours. This is an emergency situation.

Unfortunately, quite a few people ignore groin lumps, hoping they'll just go away. This is not a good idea, for two reasons:

1 It's a basic rule that any unexplained lump, anywhere in the body, requires examination by a doctor pretty soon, in order to find out what it is.

  After all, this swelling may not be due to a hernia. A number of other disorders can resemble ruptures, by causing a swelling in the groin. Some of them are relatively trivial, but others aren't. (See the section entitled 'What else could the lump be?', later in this chapter.)

2 Even if the swelling *is* due to a hernia, please bear in mind that hernias can have serious complications. Your doctor can assess the swelling, and assess the risk of those complications.

16

What is the lump like?

When you first notice the lump, it'll probably be quite small – maybe about the size of a large marble. But some ruptures are about as big as a golf ball when they're first noticed. Groin hernias are not usually very much larger than that, though occasionally one sees a lump as big as a tangerine.

In men, the lump may well find its way downwards, into the scrotum. (This is one reason why males are often embarrassed about hernias.) As we'll see a little later, there is only one particular type of groin hernia which does this.

The lump should be soft – in other words, when you prod it with your fingers, it should 'give'. Indeed, you may actually feel a bit of a bubbly sensation under your finger-tips, as a piece of intestine moves away from you with a slight gurgle.

If the lump is hard – if, when you press it, it feels like wood or stone – then you must see a doctor *immediately*. Either there's a complication of the hernia (see 'Possible complications' section in Chapter 4), or else the lump isn't due to a hernia at all.

The lump shouldn't be tender to your touch. If it is, then contact your doctor right away.

Finally, a very striking feature of many hernias is that the lump comes and goes. Sometimes you feel it – and sometimes you don't!

Other possible indications

So the commonest way of realizing that you have a rupture is by discovering a lump. But some people notice other indications before any lump appears. These include:

- Pain in the lower right-hand or left-hand corner of the abdomen. This isn't usually severe; it's more of a dull ache which comes and goes.
- Pain running down into the testicle – again, this isn't usually severe, but it's enough of an ache to be noticeable.
- A 'dragging feeling' low down in the corner of the abdomen. Dragging feelings are very hard to define – but if you keep getting a sensation like this, then you need to be checked out for a hernia.
- A feeling of weakness or of 'something giving way' in the groin region.

If you have any of the above symptoms, then you should make an appointment with your GP for an examination.

Your GP's examination

When you go to your GP because you have a groin lump, or other symptoms suggestive of a rupture, she should examine you carefully.

The correct procedure for examining a possible hernia patient is:

1 The doctor should ask you to strip off completely below the waist. Please don't be embarrassed by this – it really is necessary in order to find out precisely what the problem is.
2 She will then ask you to stand upright, and will inspect your groin to see if a lump is visible.
3 She will then ask you to cough – a request which has bewildered many patients over the years. The point of getting you to cough is that it increases the pressure inside your abdomen – which will push any hernia outwards and make it easier to see, and to feel with the finger-tips.

   Incidentally, don't be offended when the doctor asks you to turn your face away before coughing! Doctors are a lot more aware of germs than most other folk, and are not very keen on having people cough all over them.
4 The doctor will usually finish by asking you to lie on the couch to see if the swelling disappears – as is often the case with hernias. She will then feel your groin again carefully with her finger-tips, and ask you to cough several more times.

At the end of this examination, your GP should be able to tell:

• Whether you actually do have a hernia;
• What sort of groin hernia it is.

What else could the lump be?

It is a great mistake to think that any lump in the groin must be due to a hernia. Other possible causes of swelling in the groin area include:

- **Swollen glands.** The little glands in the groin frequently swell up – either as a result of some general illness, or as a reaction to some problem in either the leg or the genital area. For instance, if you happen to have an infected toe, a gland in your groin may well swell up and give the impression that you've suddenly developed a hernia.
- **Varicocoele** (pronounced VARR-ik-o-seal). This is a collection of varicose veins. It often occurs in men, and is located just above the testicle. It too can mimic a rupture.
- **Hydrocoele** (pronounced HIDE-ro-seal). This common condition in men can also mimic a hernia. It's a collection of fluid around and above the testicle.

  There is a rather similar condition in women, called 'hydrocoele of the canal of Nück'. It too is a fluid-filled swelling in the groin.
- **Lipoma.** This is a benign (harmless) fatty swelling. Lipomas may occur in many places in the body – including the groin.
- **An incompletely descended testicle.** Obviously, this is a men-only cause of groin swelling. Well before a male is born, his testicles descend from inside his belly, moving down into his scrotum. Sometimes a testicle can get stuck in the groin area during this descent; the swelling may then be mistaken for a hernia. In nearly all such cases, there is only one testicle – rather than two – in the scrotum.

From this list, it's pretty clear that diagnosing your own groin swelling as a hernia is rather a dodgy idea. Go to your own GP and let *her* make the diagnosis.

Different types of groin hernia

Life is never simple, and unfortunately there is more than one kind of groin hernia. When your doctor examines you, she will try and determine which type you have. In practice, this is not always easy: GPs find it quite difficult to differentiate between the various kinds – and even surgeons have been known to be mistaken.

Does it matter to you what kind of groin rupture you have? Not a great deal, in all honesty. But there are one or two points which you might like to know about – particularly if you are feeling a bit

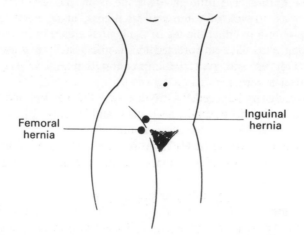

Figure 4   The two main types of groin hernia – inguinal and femoral.

doubtful about having the operation, and are considering having a truss instead. One particular type of groin hernia simply cannot be controlled by a truss.

There are two main varieties of groin hernia. They are called:

- inguinal (pronounced INN-gwyn-al);
- femoral (pronounced FEM-or-al).

Figure 4 shows that inguinal hernias occur slightly higher than femoral ones. The main difference between them is that inguinal hernias break through just above the line of the groin, while femoral ones break through just below it. Femoral hernias are more common in women than in men – but inguinal hernias are the most common type in both sexes.

Femoral hernias are particularly liable to the very serious complication called *strangulation* (which is explained in Chapter 4). In addition, femoral hernias cannot under any circumstances be controlled by trusses. Therefore, femoral hernias must always, always be operated on – and *as soon as is reasonably practicable.*

Just to complicate matters further, inguinal hernias come in two forms, called 'indirect' and 'direct'.

- **Indirect** hernias bulge downwards towards the sex organs; this is the type of hernia which, in males, may finish up by entering the scrotum.
- **Direct** hernias bulge outwards rather than diagonally downwards. This is the type of rupture which may sometimes be safely left alone (that is, not operated on), according to the guidelines of the Royal College of Surgeons of England. But this can only be done if the direct hernia is small, and 'goes back' easily.

In practice, even direct inguinal hernias are nearly always treated by surgical repair – except when the patient is old and infirm.

What happens next?

What happens next is that your GP will want you to go and see a surgeon.

There really is no sensible alternative to this. GPs do not (except in rare cases) send people to truss-makers; nor will they refer you to anybody who claims to be able to cure large holes in the groin with herbal potions. They simply send patients to the people who are experts in hernias – namely, the surgeons.

However, it's at this point that your own *choice* (if you wish to make it) may well come in – as explained in the next chapter.

4

Seeing a surgeon about a groin hernia

We've already seen that a groin hernia is a bulge which pushes its way through a small opening in your groin. And the only way to *cure* that bulge is by having surgery. But what does a surgical operation for rupture involve?

What does surgery involve?

All the various types of hernia surgery have the same aim: to push the bulge back inside your belly – and to close the hole up.

To see how this is done, let's look more closely at a hernia, and what is actually *in* the bulge. Figure 5a makes this clear. As you can see, the bulge is composed of two things:

- an outer covering;
- a central part.

The outer covering is actually the lining of your belly (medically called the 'peritoneum'). In our drawing, the central part of the hernia is a coil of intestine – but it can often be a piece of omentum – a big, fatty fold which hangs down inside your abdomen.

The obvious way to cure a hernia is shown in Figure 5b: first, the surgeon cuts through the outer covering of the bulge; then he pushes the central part of the bulge back into the belly. As you can see from Figure 5c, it's then possible to stitch the abdominal muscles together, so closing off the hole.

Another way of looking at it is to imagine that somebody's big toe is sticking out of a hole in his sock, and you have to do running repairs. You push the big toe back inside the hole – and then you darn the hole in the sock. Broadly speaking, that's what a hernia surgeon does.

However, there are now various different ways of operating – which we'll consider in Chapter 5. But first, do groin hernias really need an operation?

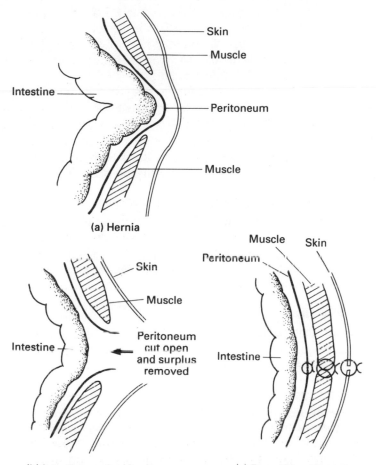

Figure 5   A hernia and its repair:
a   the composition of a hernia;
b   the peritoneum is cut open, and the surplus removed;
c   peritoneum, muscle and skin are stitched up.

Why groin hernias need surgery

There's a simple reason why most groin ruptures really do need surgery. It can be summed up in one word: *complications*. Unfortunately a hernia which is left uncured can often run into big trouble – complications of hernias are common. They're particularly frequent with femoral hernias (described in Chapter 3). So if you know that you have a femoral hernia, you should do everything in your power to make sure that you get operated on *as soon as possible* – in case complications occur.

What causes complications? It's quite simple really. Imagine your hernia as a swelling roughly the size of a small pear; then imagine that it has passed through a hole which is about the size of a wedding ring. Clearly, there's a great danger that the hernia will be constricted or 'nipped' at the point where it passes through that fairly narrow hole. If this happens, then complications are likely.

Possible complications if surgery is avoided

So what are these complications which may arise if surgery is avoided? If you're easily upset, just skip the following list altogether! But be assured that anybody who reads about these major complications will be in no doubt that the average hernia needs an operation.

1 Irreducibility

This means that the hernia will not go back. In the early stages, most ruptures can be persuaded to slip back inside the belly – by using such manoeuvres as lying down, or pressing the bulge back inside with the fingers.

However, there often comes a point when the swelling simply cannot be induced to pop back inside the small opening in the groin – which leaves you with a permanent lump in your groin. This in itself is not a disaster, though the ever-present lump may be unsightly (it's sometimes visible through the clothes). Also, the lump may now be quite uncomfortable, or even painful.

But the really important aspect of an irreducible hernia is that, because the lump will not go back, there is a risk of the more serious complications of obstruction or strangulation (see next two sections).

Therefore, when a hernia becomes irreducible, it's a strong indication that it's high time you had an operation on it.

2 Obstruction

If there is intestine (gut or bowel) trapped inside the hernia, then it is very easy for intestinal obstruction to occur. In other words, your intestines become blocked, so that nothing can get through. This is

24

really serious, and you will become ill very quickly. Symptoms of intestinal blockage include:

- pain in the abdomen;
- inability to pass bowel motions or even wind;
- vomiting.

An emergency operation to relieve the obstruction is necessary.

3 Strangulation

An untreated hernia may become strangulated – that is, the blood supply to it may become 'nipped off' at the narrow opening in the groin. If this happens, the potential for disaster is very great. I have seen several people die as a result of neglected hernias which became strangulated.

Symptoms of a strangulated hernia include:

- pain of quite sudden onset, over the area of the hernia;
- within a few hours, generalized abdominal pain;
- forcible and repeated vomiting.

If the diagnosis is not made promptly, and the patient is not taken to hospital for an emergency operation, gangrene usually sets in within a few hours.

I trust that this rather alarming account has made it very clear that one of the major reasons for operating on a hernia is to avoid strangulation at all costs.

Terms explained

Finally, there are a couple of potentially confusing terms which are used when talking about complications of ruptures – terms which need explanation:

- **Incarcerated hernia.** You may hear the term 'incarcerated hernia' – a phrase which unfortunately has different meanings in different countries. In Britain, it generally means much the same thing as 'obstructed' (see above), and often implies that there are bowel motions trapped within the hernia.

  However, in the USA and some other countries, the expression 'incarceration' is often used more loosely to mean either strangulation or obstruction.

- **Richter's hernia** (also called **Richter's strangulated hernia**). This is a complication in which only a small part of the bowel – not the whole width of it – is trapped in the hole in the groin. The early symptoms are not usually as severe as those of ordinary strangulation. But a prompt diagnosis, followed by an emergency operation, may be life-saving.

Getting to see a surgeon

After your GP has diagnosed a hernia, you need to see a surgeon soon, in order to have it assessed.

When it comes to seeing a surgeon, some element of *choice* comes in – though to be frank, there's much more choice if you have private medical insurance, or can afford private fees.

Though there has been a great increase in private surgery in recent years, the great majority of hernia patients in Britain will go through the long-established NHS route, as shown on the top line of our flow chart (Figure 6). When your GP has seen you, she writes a letter to a surgeon at an NHS hospital, and you'll then be sent an appointment to see the surgeon – after a variable period of waiting.

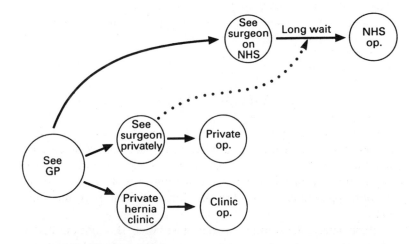

Figure 6 The routes to surgery, on the NHS and privately.

I wish I could say that the wait to see the surgeon will be short, but in many parts of the country it just isn't. For instance, in the region where I work, it can be anything between two and six months. So it's a good idea to ask your GP how long it might take to get to see each of the NHS surgeons in your area. She should be able to find this out, because in most parts of the UK, GPs are sent regularly updated lists of waiting times.

However, don't make the mistake of thinking that the surgeon with the shortest waiting time is the one you should necessarily go for. Ideally, what you need is the surgeon with the most expertise in hernia surgery.

You might think that all surgeons are equally good at all operations – but you would be wrong. So ask your GP to say which surgeon she thinks would be best. If by any chance she doesn't really know, then it would be worth your while asking around locally, among people who've had hernia operations before you make up your mind.

One small additional point: these days, it's very common to go into your GP's surgery and see a locum (temporary) doctor. He's not very likely to know a lot about the local surgeons, so it may be better to make a further appointment, in order to chat the matter over with your own regular GP.

With luck, your doctor may know whether any of the NHS surgeons in the area are doing the new-style hernia operations (described fully in Chapter 5). These operations are associated with a very much quicker recovery time than is the case with traditional hernia repair.

NHS or private?

As we've just seen, you can wait a very long time to see an NHS surgeon about your hernia. (Admittedly, if your rupture is causing you a lot of trouble, or if it is of a type which is particularly liable to complications, your GP may well be willing to write a letter asking for your appointment to be brought forward. This may do some good.)

Unfortunately, the waiting has only just begun. It's not until after you've seen the surgeon that you get on to the hospital admission list. And – despite attempts to shorten them – these lists are often outrageously long. In the past, I have seen hernia patients having to wait for almost two years for surgery. And even today, a wait of many months is common.

So it is not surprising that large numbers of people decide to go privately. If you disapprove on moral grounds, then clearly this route isn't for you. But if you have private medical insurance, then obviously, you are unlikely to bother with going through the NHS. The fact is that these days, many men and women who haven't got medical insurance do nevertheless choose to see a surgeon privately – and often go on to have the operation privately as well.

You can see this route on the middle line of our flow chart (Figure 6). In most cases, paying for a private consultation will get you to see a surgeon very quickly indeed. You're unlikely to have to wait more than a couple of weeks, unless the surgeon's private practice is very large, or he is away on holiday! There are a few places where you'd be no quicker going privately to a surgeon than seeing him under the NHS – but they are pretty rare.

You may like to note that it's often possible just to *consult* a surgeon privately – but then to go on and have the operation under the NHS, at his NHS hospital. Some health authorities don't like you doing this, but it is a possibility. That route is shown by the dotted line on Figure 6.

Does that enable you to jump the queue? Unfortunately this did sometimes happen in the old days. A surgeon would see a patient privately – and the patient would then mysteriously appear towards the top of his NHS waiting list, and be admitted very shortly to hospital! That kind of thing is totally and utterly wrong: the authorities are supposed to have stamped on it, and it should not occur nowadays.

If you look at the lowest part of Figure 6, you'll see that there is now another route – to go to a private hernia clinic. As explained in Chapter 1, these specialist hernia centres have sprung up in the last few years. They don't do any other operations except hernia repairs, and you get seen quickly – and operated on quickly.

Also, they almost invariably use the new-style operations (such as the mesh repair – see Chapter 5), so that patients can be discharged on the day they have surgery. The operation is normally done under local anaesthetic, rather than a general anaesthetic.

Private hernia centres now advertise widely in the newspapers and on radio. They compete with each other, and this arguably helps to keep costs down (see 'Costs of private surgery', below). Under present legislation – which will probably change – it's sometimes possible for a private clinic to do your operation under the NHS, if your GP is a fund holder.

Advantages and disadvantages of going privately

There are clearly certain advantages and disadvantages to going privately:

Advantages

* You will almost certainly be seen by a surgeon more quickly;
* You will almost certainly be operated on more quickly;
* You can have the operation when *you* choose to have it;
* Although there's sometimes a reluctance to admit this fact, the
  - chances are that you will be dealt with in a more considered and unhurried fashion – and in more comfortable circumstances than the NHS can afford;
* You can be sure of who your surgeon is – in other words, you can be certain that he will not delegate the operation to a junior.

Disadvantages

* It will cost you a lot of money (see below), unless you have private medical insurance;
* The care in some small private hospitals is frankly not very good – especially if things start going wrong.

Costs of private surgery

If you are considering paying for your treatment yourself (rather than having an insurance company pay it for you), it's important to remember that you are entering a market-place! So there are no rules to limit what a surgeon may charge you for an initial private consultation: in general, they charge what the market will bear.

At the present time, you may well find that a surgeon working in the provinces charges anything between £50 and £100 for a consultation. But in the ritzier parts of London, a fashionable consultant might well ask for much more than that. The only safe rule is to ask his secretary *beforehand* what his charges will be. (Curiously enough, I find that British patients are very reluctant to do this – they mistakenly think that it is impolite to ask about costs.)

Bear in mind that, if the initial consultation reveals the need for

29

any laboratory tests or X-rays, the expense of having these done could be considerable. In practice, most hernia patients do not need such investigations.

What about the costs of the actual operation? Here again, you are in a market-place – and a fairly expensive one at that. There is no law which says what a surgeon may charge for a hernia operation – nor is there one governing what the anaesthetist may charge, or what the hospital may bill you for (theatre time, nursing care and drugs are all expensive).

To give you an idea of the wide disparity of charges: at the present time it is possible to pay as little as £800 and as much as £4,000 for a hernia repair operation in the UK. So once again, if you're going to pay the bill yourself, ask *beforehand* about the charges – preferably getting the figure in writing.

Private hernia centres, which provide a standard package, should be perfectly open and up-front about what they are charging. At the present time, the two best-known such clinics in Britain are quoting a price of about £900 for a straightforward hernia operation by the mesh method. (See also Useful Addresses at the end of this book.)

Your interview with the surgeon

But whether you choose to go on the NHS or privately, there will come a day when you have an appointment with the surgeon. He will examine you, decide precisely what type of hernia you've got, make an assessment of how urgently it needs to be operated on – and then tell you what he proposes to do.

Now this interview is of great importance to you, and you should make the most of it. This will be a lot easier if you are seeing the consultant privately, since you are paying for his time – and you will get quite a lot of it! I wish I could say that you'll get plenty of time with the specialist if you see him on the NHS, but that is unlikely to prove true.

However, even if you're seeing the surgeon on the NHS, you should try and make sure that all your questions are answered by him. Regrettably, my post-bag shows that quite often the patient does not get much in the way of answers. The medical profession likes to present itself as approachable and sympathetic – and very frequently that's just what it is. But I have to be honest and say that many consultant surgeons are desperately hard-pressed for time – and rather brusque. Unfortunately, the spirit of the surgeon who was played by James Robertson Justice in the film *Doctor in the House* is not entirely dead. I'm sorry to say that I've seen surgeons examine a patient and then bark out: 'You've got a rupture there. We'll put you on the waiting list. Good morning.' Exit surgeon!

On the other hand, nowadays there *are* many nice, friendly, caring, communicative consultant surgeons – who really do take the trouble to sit down and talk things over with you properly. But if your consultant isn't like that, and you can't get him to answer your questions fully and clearly, then your best move is to ask one of his staff to clarify things for you. Grab his senior registrar or other assisting doctor, and make sure you get answers! After all, it's your body.

Questions you should always ask

There are certain things you should *always* ask the surgeon, or one of his staff. However, these days there's an increasing tendency for patients to be given helpful leaflets which explain a lot about the procedure they're being booked in for. Such a leaflet may well answer a lot of your queries, but you will probably also have other questions in mind.

Here are some of the questions which you should obtain answers to before you leave the clinic:

- 'Which kind of operation are you going to use? A traditional darning-type repair, or one of the new procedures like the mesh operation or keyhole surgery?'

  If the reply is that the surgeon is going to use the old, traditional method, it's worth asking why – since the procedure does take quite a time to recover from. However, it may well be the right one for you.
- 'What is the likelihood that a testicle will have to be removed during surgery?'

  If you feel strongly about this, Chapters 6 and 9 cover it more fully.
- 'If you're going to use one of the new operations on me, what are the results like in your unit? And how long have you been doing it?'

  Many British patients feel that this sort of question is too

31

cheeky to ask. Yet, as we'll see in Chapter 5, there can be very real dangers when a surgeon unwisely undertakes a new operation with which he's unfamiliar.

• 'What's the chance of recurrence of my hernia after your operation?'

This really is a 64,000-dollar question. Most people don't realize that many ruptures do recur within a few years of undergoing surgery – just as if that old darned sock had given way again! So ask your surgeon or his assistant what the likelihood of this is.

• 'Are you going to do the operation under general anaesthetic – or local?'

Only a minority of ruptures are dealt with under local anaesthetic – but the proportion is increasing, particularly as the new day-case mesh operation becomes more common.

• 'How long will it be before I can go home/drive the car/work/ make love?'

The answers will vary greatly, depending on the surgeon, the hospital, and what kind of operation you're going to have. But at this stage, somebody ought to be able to give you an accurate estimation.

• 'How long am I going to be on the waiting list?'

Don't be fobbed off on this one. Somebody should at least be able to tell you whether the current waiting list is weeks long – or months long. They should also tell you how much notice you'll get when you're summoned for admission.

What to do while you're on the waiting list

If you're on a private waiting list, it will be very short indeed; it will be surprising if you're not in hospital within a couple of weeks. On the NHS, however, you will almost certainly have to wait quite a bit longer. At least this will give you a bit of time to reflect – and to change your mind if you wish (see below).

During this period, if you have any worries or queries – or even if you feel like going to another surgeon – you should talk things over with your GP. She should be able to resolve any concerns you may have.

Incidentally, don't make the common mistake of going to see her just a few days after consulting the surgeon. At this stage, she will not yet have received the all-important letter from the hospital, giving the surgeon's opinion and saying what he is planning to do. So wait for a week or two, till the consultant has had plenty of time to write to your GP.

Preparing yourself for the operation

Is there anything you can do for yourself while you're on the waiting list? Yes, there is: it's well worth trying to get into the best possible shape for the operation. Here are some useful tips:

- If you're overweight, try to slim down. This will ease the pressure inside your abdomen, and so help to prevent the hernia from getting worse. It will also make the operation easier for the surgeons. And – most important – it will probably reduce your chances of a recurrence (the rupture returning after the operation).
- If you're a smoker, give up. If you can't give up, then cut down. This will make you a better 'operation risk'. It will also reduce the chances of post-operative coughing – which can contribute to a recurrence.
- Try and get your abdominal muscles in shape. The muscles in the region of the rupture are often weak, thin and out of condition. Anything you can reasonably do to help them become stronger and bulkier will make the operation easier – and reduce the chances of recurrence. You don't necessarily have to go down to the gym and work out. But sensible exercise, like walking – coupled perhaps with a few daily sit-ups – will tone up those muscles, and do you a lot of good.
- If by any chance you are taking the contraceptive pill, then you will probably have to discontinue it for at least a fortnight before your operation, in order to reduce the risk of getting blood clots. Your GP or Family Planning Clinic can help you with the timing of this, so that you don't run any risks of unwanted pregnancy.

Changing your mind

During your time on the waiting list, you do at least have the opportunity of changing your mind if you want to. I can remember a number of patients who did this during the long months of waiting.

Stephen, in his early 30s, found that his rupture was seriously impairing his ability to work – and also impairing his earnings. His GP couldn't get him moved up the waiting list.

So he went to his bank manager, got a loan, and saw a surgeon privately. His hernia was operated on a week later – and he was back at full earning-power within a few weeks.

Roger, in his late 70s, decided that he didn't really want to face going through with the operation. After discussion with his GP and with an understanding surgeon, he was referred to an orthotist (the expert who fits the surgical appliances at a hospital). He was measured up for a truss, which controlled his particular hernia very satisfactorily for many years.

Valerie, a businesswoman in her 40s, lived in a part of the country where only the traditional hernia repair, with its long post-operative recovery time, was on offer. She wasn't looking forward to being off work for weeks after surgery.

So, after hearing a radio commercial, she went to a hernia centre where she had one of the newer operations done as a day case. It went very well, and she was fortunate in being able to get back to light work within a few days.

In the next chapter, we shall move on to look at the various possible forms of surgery – including the new ones.

5

Types of surgery for groin hernias

This chapter looks at the various kinds of surgery which may be used in order to repair your groin rupture.

If you're the sort of person who says, 'The doctors know best – I'll leave it all to them', then fine: this chapter is not for you! But if you want to know what the options are so that you can exercise some choice (if possible), then this chapter describes the pros and cons of the various methods – including the ones that are currently being so widely advertised to the public.

A climate of change

It's important to understand that things have changed very fast in the field of hernia repair during the last few years.

The traditional operation for groin rupture was invented in late Victorian days. For about 100 years, virtually everybody who underwent hernia surgery had this type of operation. Unfortunately, there's a certain amount of pain afterwards, and it takes quite a long time to achieve full recovery. So surgeons started looking around for new procedures, and several of these came into widespread use during the 1990s.

The new operations do however have their plus and minus points – the most important minus point being that, as they've been in use for such a short time, we don't really know what the long-term results will be.

In addition, in many parts of the British Isles, it is as yet very difficult to obtain anything other than the traditional operation; if you want to try one of the new alternatives, you may well have to travel in order to get it.

Also, the new procedures are at present mainly done privately; most NHS hernia repairs are still done by the traditional method. But that will change.

My own feeling is that if you want to try and make an intelligent choice about what sort of operation you could have, you should read this chapter – and then talk things over with your GP. You can also obtain further information from the addresses which are given at the end of this book.

Traditional surgery

To all intents and purposes, the traditional operation to repair a hernia was invented by the great Italian surgeon Bassini, in about 1880. There are many variations on it, depending partly on which type of groin hernia you have – but from the patient's point of view, they all come down to much the same thing.

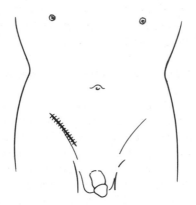

Figure 7   The location of a traditional hernia operation.

The surgeon makes a cut 7 to 10 centimetres (3/4 inches) long, at approximately the location shown in Figure 7. This means that after your skin has healed up you will have a small scar of that length.

The surgeon can then get at the bulge, push it back inside your abdomen – and set to work to repair the hole through which it came. By skilful stitching, he can close the gap almost completely, leaving only enough space for certain important structures, like blood-carrying tubes, which pass through the little apertures in the groin (as shown in Figure 2). The fact that these gaps cannot be completely closed is one reason why hernias can recur.

The traditional operation is most often done under general

36

anaesthetic. These days, however, there's an increasing tendency to carry it out under a local anaesthetic – especially if the patient has a bad chest or is otherwise a bad risk for a general. You'll find details about how you'll feel after the operation, and how long it will take you to recover, in Chapters 6 and 7.

Note: variants of the traditional repair are known by such names as McArthur's operation, the Canadian (Shouldice) repair, and – for femoral hernias only – Lotheissen's repair.

The mesh operation

You may well have seen newspaper adverts or heard radio commercials which extol the merits of the mesh operation (also called 'open mesh procedure'). The publicity claims that it's superior to the traditional operation, that there's very little pain, and that you will be back to work in no time. All such adverts should be taken with a pinch of salt – nevertheless, there is a lot to be said for this operation.

The open mesh procedure is an operation, almost invariably done under local anaesthetic, in which the surgeon makes a small incision in your groin, pushes back the hernia and then repairs the hole by simply sewing in a mesh 'patch'. This patch is slightly larger than the side of a matchbox, and it can be made of various materials – polypropylene being currently the most common.

Once the mesh has been fixed in place, the surgeon closes up and that's it. The whole process usually takes much less than an hour, making it considerably shorter than the traditional operation.

The great advantage of the mesh procedure is that it avoids the deep, 'darning' stitches which are used in the older operation. There's absolutely no doubt that you have less pain afterwards, and that you are likely to make a very fast recovery, and be back to work quickly. Patients generally like it, because they can be on their feet – or even riding an exercise bike – within an hour or two of the operation.

Surgeons who do the open mesh procedure say that complication rates are low, and that very few people suffer recurrence of their ruptures.

However, the mesh operation in its present form is still relatively new. As with any innovation in medicine, it will take some years to assess it fully. There's always an outside chance that, in the years to come, it will turn out that open mesh surgery can have unsuspected drawbacks – like (perhaps) a surprisingly high recurrence rate.

But for the moment, the prospects for mesh surgery look good, and the number of surgeons who are using it is increasing. It is highly significant that the private hernia centres are making so much use of it.

For details about recovery and self-care after having an open mesh operation, see Chapters 6 and 7.

Keyhole (laparoscopic) hernia repair

The phrase 'keyhole surgery' means that the surgeon operates through very tiny incisions, while seeing what she is doing by looking through a slim, telescope-like device called a laparoscope – which is why the other name for this procedure is laparoscopic surgery.

The great beauty of keyhole surgery is that the surgeons do not have to cut you open to see what's going on inside. They can get a good view simply by looking through the eyepiece – though these days, the instrument is usually connected to a TV monitor in the operating theatre.

Laparoscopic surgery has proved wonderfully valuable in certain fields, particularly gynaecology and the treatment of knee injuries. Because the patients have such very small incisions, they recover very much fast faster – and with much less pain.

But not everything is marvellous about keyhole surgery. The Press have hailed it as though it were a miracle – but it's important to realize that it can go spectacularly wrong. You should be aware of this before deciding to choose this method of having your hernia repaired.

Why can it go wrong? In short, because the surgeon is looking at a *two*-dimensional picture – not a three-dimensional one. When you gaze at a TV screen, you have no accurate perception of depth – and a surgeon who operates laparoscopically cannot accurately perceive depth either. This does not matter if he has been very carefully trained to carry out keyhole surgery – but in the early days of various laparoscopic procedures, a lot of mistakes were made. Some patients were damaged, and ended up suing their surgeons.

These days, mistakes should not happen, since operators are

supposed to go on special courses in which they practise using the keyhole instruments on 'dummy' patients. But unfortunately not all consultants are sensible enough to undertake that kind of specialist training. In the mid-1990s, a very well-known London gynaecologist was struck off the medical register by the General Medical Council for recklessly damaging patients during laparoscopic surgery; he had believed that he was too clever to need supervision or training.

Having said all that, I would like to reassure you that if a surgeon offers to repair your hernia by keyhole surgery, privately or otherwise – the odds are that he will be highly skilled and experienced in the technique. None the less, if I were the patient, I'd certainly ask him how many cases he'd done, and what his results were. At the present time, there are only a few dozen British consultants who are curing hernias by laparoscopic surgery. Some are working under the NHS, and some privately.

Most patients have day-case surgery – that is, they go home the same day. Nearly all of them have a general anaesthetic, but it's possible that local anaesthesia may be used more in the years to come. The operation takes about 45 to 60 minutes.

What happens is that, once you're asleep, the surgeon makes three tiny nicks in the skin of your lower abdomen. The telescope-like device is pushed through one of these, and instruments are passed through the other two (one instrument for each hand).

On the TV minitor, the surgeon should now be able to see the *inside* of the hole through which your hernia has pushed. He uses his instruments to repair the gap, often inserting the type of mesh used in the open mesh operation (see above). Having done this, he withdraws the instruments and the viewing device. The three little cuts are so small that you may not need any stitches – just three elastoplasts or Band-Aids. (This is why in the USA, laparoscopy is often known as 'Band-Aid surgery'.)

Having had such tiny incisions, you should recover very quickly. A surgeon who is one of the leading exponents of this method told me that the results are good, and that complications are rare. He thinks this is 'the method of the future'.

However, it's rather early days yet, and a recent Royal College of Surgeons report suggested that it would be some years before we could fully assess the place of keyhole surgery in the treatment of ruptures. As with any new method, it will be at least 15 years before the risk of recurrence is known.

For details of recovery and self-care after laparoscopy, please see Chapters 6 and 7.

The plug method

In the second half of the 1990s, there has suddenly been a great deal of publicity for an entirely new method of treating groin hernias: the 'plug' method. It originated in America, but has recently been energetically promoted in Britain and elsewhere.

The basic idea is that, having made a small incision in your groin, the surgeon blocks up the hernia hole with a plug made of synthetic material. The plug (marketed under the name 'PerFix') looks remarkably like the head of a flower. The intention is that its 'petals' will expand, neatly filling up the hole in your groin.

From the patient's point of view, a major advantage of the plug method is that the operation is very short: it takes only 20 minutes or so. At the clinic in the USA where the method was developed, people are allowed to go home just 90 minutes after getting off the operating table. As a rule, a general anaesthetic is unnecessary – the Americans use a type of regional anaesthetic called an epidural (in which the numbing agent is injected at the base of the spine).

Advocates of the PerFix plug are currently making enthusiastic claims for its patient-acceptability, and the low infection rate apparently associated with it. But it's *very* early days with this particular method, and it will be far into the twenty-first century before anyone really knows the long-term rates of recurrence of the hernia.

Assessing the various types of surgery

In summary, these days you may be able to choose between four different methods of surgery:

- The traditional repair – which is still the method most widely practised in the NHS;
- The mesh (or open mesh) procedure – which is widely available in private clinics, but is spreading into the NHS;
- The keyhole (or laparoscopic) method – which is at present only available on a small scale, both in the NHS and privately;

- The plug technique – which at the moment is carried out by only a handful of British surgeons.

Where you have a choice, you may well be influenced by the fact that the newer operations (the mesh procedure, the plug technique, and the keyhold method) are very suitable for day surgery – and patients recover very fast from them. However, I cannot over-emphasize the fact that we don't yet know for certain what the risk of recurrence is with the newer techniques.

Recurrence

Recurrence is a word which every rupture patient should bear in mind. Most people haven't the faintest notion that many hernia operations fail – in other words, the rupture eventually reappears. Even with the traditional method of surgery, the risk of recurrence is quite high: surgical textbooks quote rates of between 5 per cent and 15 per cent. If we accept that 10 per cent is about average, then this means that one in 10 of all those who have hernia operations will find that their ruptures come back again.

When this happens, it's no joke – because it may not be possible to do a second repair-job on the hernia (think of it as trying to redarn a sock which is getting more and more worn and frayed). So some people whose rupture has recurred end up having to use a truss instead of having repeat surgery.

Therefore, there's a lot to be said for choosing an operation which has a low recurrence rate. I have spoken to surgeons who claim that the recurrence rates with the newer operations are 'only one to two per cent'. If this proves to be true, it will be great. But at the moment, it's still very much a case of 'if'.

The future

There is no doubt that the early years of the twenty-first century will see interesting new developments in hernia treatment – probably involving the development of devices (made out of synthetic material) to block the hole in the groin which, as we've seen, is the root cause of all ruptures in this region.

But whatever new method of hernia therapy you are offered, I hope you will bear in mind the points which have been emphasized in this chapter:

- How long has the surgeon been doing it?
- What is the recurrence rate?

Chapter 6 explains what exactly happens to you when you go into hospital.

6

Going into hospital

Day-case surgery

These days, many people with hernias are treated on what's called a 'day-case basis' – in other words, they come into hospital in the morning, have the operation done, and then go home that night.

Nearly all open mesh repairs and keyhole surgery repairs are done in this way. And an increasing number of traditional hernia repairs are also being carried out this way. However, the traditional-style operation does still very often involve staying a few nights in hospital; that type of in-patient surgery will be dealt with in the second part of this chapter.

Preparation for going in

The hospital or clinic will probably send you a leaflet telling you what they want you to do before you come in for day-case surgery. Obviously, you need to follow the advice in this leaflet, but it will probably give advice along these lines:

- If you're going to have a general anaesthetic, don't have anything to eat or drink for at least eight hours before the operation. (Very often, this means having nothing after about midnight.) Please do follow this guideline strictly. To have *anything* in your stomach when you are given a general anaesthetic may well cause vomiting – and that can even be fatal, since it may induce choking.
- Do not have alcohol the night before your operation.
- If you're on any medication, bring it with you to the hospital so that the medical staff can see what it is.
- It's usually a good idea to try and have a morning bowel motion before setting off for the hospital. Some surgeons will want you to use a suppository the night before the operation.
- To prevent infection, it's essential that the hair in the region of the operation is shaved off. In the old days, this was often done by a member of the hospital staff shortly before surgery. Nowadays, it's likely that you'll be asked to do it yourself the night before. The hospital or clinic will tell you how much needs to be removed.

Admission for day-case surgery

When you're going to have day-case surgery, it's a good idea to get to the hospital or clinic in plenty of time, so that you arrive feeling fresh and unflustered. Rushing pushes your blood pressure up, which is not generally a good idea.

It may seem a minor point, but it's worth remembering that the parking at many hospitals is absolutely dreadful in the mornings these days. You don't want to spend half an hour desperately searching for a parking slot, or trying to get change for the machine. In fact, there is much to be said for either taking a taxi, or getting a friend or relative to drive you in.

Don't take any valuables (credit cards, jewellery, etc.) with you. Sadly, security in hospitals is a major problem, so it is best to take in no more than a pound or two – just in case you want to make some small purchase later in the day. You needn't really take any belongings with you at all, unless you want to have something (toiletries, make-up) with which to tidy yourself up before you go home later in the day.

You'll find that with day-case surgery there are very few formalities, and the whole process is very speedy. One thing you will have to deal with, however, is the consent form.

The consent form

Before undergoing day-case surgery – or any other type of surgery, for that matter – you need to sign a consent form. This is not a legal requirement: it's simply that the surgeons and the hospital or clinic require it for their own protection. No surgeon in his right mind will operate on you unless a consent form has been signed, because this would leave him open to being sued.

There's a sample consent form in the second part of this chapter (which is about in-patient surgery).

One final tip: read the consent form carefully *before* you have any pre-medication, and make sure that you're signing for the operation which you intend to undergo. *After* you've had pre-medication, you may well be a little woozy and have difficulty in understanding any unclear wording.

Day-case surgery under local anaesthetic

A good deal of day-case hernia surgery is done under *local* anaesthetic. Indeed, at the present time, virtually all open mesh operations are being carried out under local anaesthesia. (At the moment, nearly all keyhole surgery and most traditional-type hernia repairs are done under general.)

I think that having a local anaesthetic is really very good, because you don't have any of the risks associated with general anaesthesia. You can lie there peacefully, and talk to the surgeon if you want to – and in many operating theatres these days, you can listen to music. Some people do flinch at the idea of a local anaesthetic, but in fact it's nothing to be worried about. The odds are that you'll feel nothing more than a slight jab at the beginning – and that's it.

There are various ways in which the local anaesthesia may be given, but a common one is for the surgeon to inject a small amount of a numbing solution into the skin of your belly. Once that patch of skin has 'deadened' (which will take only a minute or two), he can move on from there, injecting more local anaesthetic as he goes – the likelihood is that you won't be able to feel a thing.

Warning: One very minor problem with a local anaesthetic is that it may make your leg 'give way' in the hours immediately after the operation. This is nothing to worry about – it's just that the nerves are still partly numbed. But for the first 12 hours after you leave the hospital or clinic, you should be very careful about climbing stairs or getting in and out of cars.

Under no circumstances should you drive yourself home, since there is a chance that you might not be able to control the pedals properly.

Day-case surgery under a general anaesthetic

A lot of day-case hernia surgery is done under general anaesthesia, including virtually all keyhole surgery and many traditional-type rupture repairs.

If you *are* given a general anaesthetic, it will be a 'light' one, from which you should wake up reasonably briskly. You should be pretty clear-headed within an hour or so of coming round. However, don't even consider driving, going back to work, or making any important decisions that day! Your body will still contain a lot of anaesthetic drugs, which will only gradually disappear over the next couple of days.

When you come round from the operation, you may or may not feel some pain in the groin which has been operated on. If it's troubling you, tell the nurses and they will get you a painkiller.

Going home the same evening

Whether you've had a local or a general anaesthetic, you shouldn't drive. Either get a friend or relative to pick you up, or else order a taxi. Public transport is not a great idea – you need to go home in comfort, without people jammed against you.

Before you go home, a nurse or doctor should:

- See that you're not in excessive pain;
- Make sure that you've got painkilling pills to take with you (ensure you've got enough to last for several days – it's frustrating to have to drag down to your GP to get a further prescription);
- Give you a certificate for work if you need one;
- Check your operation site, making sure that the dressing is OK and not leaking;
- Tell you when the surgeon will want to see you again.

Very importantly, you should take with you *a note from the hospital or clinic to your own doctor.* If you get any problems during the next few days (which is admittedly unlikely), your GP is the one who'll have to sort them out. And if she hasn't got any written notification of exactly what the hospital has done, that makes life rather difficult for her.

So, by the evening of the day of the operation, you will be back home. What you need now is to lie down and put your feet up! Resist any temptation to do any work, or cleaning or cooking. *You must rest.* In fact, there's a lot to be said for going straight to bed, so that you keep warm, cosy and comfortable.

As far as food goes, you can eat whatever you like, but a light meal is probably best. Alcohol is best avoided this particular evening, because of the fact that the anaesthetic drugs – which don't go well with drink – are circulating in your system. Do not do what I once did after day-case surgery (on my knee), and go out to dinner. You'll probably end up falling asleep in the middle of it. Your best plan is to have an early night with a nice cup of cocoa or whatever.

A few practical points:

- The toilet: you should be able to pass water without difficulty. And if you want to have a bowel action, there's no reason why you shouldn't. However, in practice, many people don't pass any motions for a day or two.

46

- Sleep: you should be able to get a decent night's sleep after the operation. However, if pain is keeping you awake, don't hesitate to take the painkillers which you've been given. But read the label, and make sure you don't exceed the maximum dose. If you normally take a sleeping pill (which is unusual these days), you may be able to take it as well as the painkiller. But check this with the hospital or clinic before you leave for home.
- Bleeding: a slight blood loss from the operation site is perfectly normal. It is most unlikely that you will lose any significant amount of blood. But if you're worried that bleeding is more than you'd expected, ring the hospital or clinic for advice. If they have closed down for the night – which is likely in the case of a private unit – then either ring your GP or else go to the Accident & Emergency unit at your local hospital.

  First aid tip: while heavy bleeding after a day-case hernia operation is most uncommon, it's worth knowing that a good way of controlling it is to press a thick pad – e.g. a wad of cotton wool or a sanitary towel – over the bleeding point *and keep pressing continuously.*
- Sex: younger patients do sometimes consider having sex on the same night as they arrive home from a day-case operation – perhaps to prove to themselves that they still can. There's absolutely no reason why you shouldn't do this if you want to – but you should avoid violent physical activity, as you don't want to tear your stitches.

Chapter 7 gives details about looking after yourself during the few weeks that follow your operation.

In-patient surgery

Even today, a very large number of groin hernias are *not* dealt with on a day-case basis, and you have to be admitted to hospital for your operation. I say 'even today' because there has been an enormous reduction in the amount of time spent in hospital in recent years, and this reduction seems to be continuing. Hernia patients who would once have spent 11 or 12 days on the ward are now out in a day or two.

None the less, if you have the traditional-style hernia repair, the odds are that you will stay in hospital for a few nights. So this part of the chapter explains what happens to you if you're admitted as an in-patient.

Admission as an in-patient

It's a good idea to ask someone to bring you to the hospital to be admitted. Take a small suitcase or overnight bag with you, so that he can take your outdoor clothes home once you've changed into your pyjamas. (There's very little space in hospital, so unless you're in a private room you're unlikely to have room to store your day clothes.)

Things to take in with you

Here are some suggestions for things you might need while you're on the ward:

- washing kit
- shaving kit
- make-up
- notepad, envelopes, stamps
- pen
- comb and brush
- nail-file
- diary
- list of friends' and family phone numbers
- coins (and possibly cards) for the phone
- fruit squash and fruit
- pyjamas or nightie
- slippers
- dressing gown
- hankies
- glasses
- mirror
- sanitary pads or tampons
- books and magazines

If you're fond of music, it may well be worthwhile taking in a small Walkman-type radio or cassette with earphones, in case the hospital radio set-up isn't to your taste.

Note that there are no valuables on the above list. It is safer these days to bring in only a few pounds with you, and I do not recommend bringing in credit cards or jewellery (you won't be able to wear the latter in the operating theatre).

The admission procedure

These days, the actual procedure of admission is usually quite a bit simpler than it used to be. Somebody will write down a great many details, including your date of birth, postcode, telephone number and so on.

Most importantly, do let the admitting staff know what medication you're on (if any). It's helpful to bring a list of your drugs written on a piece of paper – or you could just take all the pills in with you, so that their names can be copied down from the label. Don't do what so many people do and just say, 'I'm on the brown ones – *you* know.' They *don't* know.

If you happen to be on the contraceptive pill, you should say so. As mentioned earlier, this should have been discontinued at least a fortnight before your admission, to reduce the risk of post-operative blood clots.

Also, please tell the admitting staff about any allergies you may have – not allergies to insects or grass, but allergies to things they might inadvertently prescribe for you (like penicillin) or put on your skin (like sticking plaster).

Once the clerical details have been dealt with and you've been allotted a bed, somebody will probably come round and do some basic tests; this may be a nurse or a junior doctor or both. These tests include:

- pulse rate
- blood pressure
- weight
- urine test

In NHS hospitals, a younger doctor (a house surgeon) now does what's called 'clerking you in'. This may strike you as a bit of a nuisance, but in fact it's a very good idea – because this junior doctor may well pick up important things which haven't yet been noticed.

She will ask you to recount the story of how you noticed your hernia, how much trouble it's causing you, and so on. You'll also be asked about any past illnesses you've had, and whether there are any diseases which run in your family.

The house surgeon will then give you a complete physical examination. If she finds anything which doesn't seem right – for instance if you appear pale or have signs of a chest infection – then some tests will be ordered. Common ones include:

- Blood tests: usually to check if you are anaemic (that is, if your blood count is low) – but there are many other blood tests.
- Chest X-ray: if there's any suggestion that you have a problem with your lungs.
- ECG (known in the USA and many other countries as EKG): an electrocardiograph, or electrical test on the heart. Often done on the over-50s, or on anyone with a history of chest pain.

In private hospitals, it's unlikely that a doctor will come round and give you a full physical examination. However, the anaesthetist may pop in, ask you a few questions about your health, and check your heart and lungs.

Ward life

Curiously enough, you'll probably remember your hospital stay for the rest of your life – because the experiences which people have while on a hospital ward tend to make a very big impact on them.

Not everyone enjoys being confined to hospital. In particular, if you're a person who values privacy and solitude, you might find it quite difficult – and it could be worth your while asking if you can have a side-room, or if you can go in a side-ward with only a few people in it. On the other hand, there are plenty of folk who really enjoy ward life, and who like the camaraderie of being in contact with other patients, chatting to them about their illnesses, helping to bring round the tea and so on.

Ward rules

In nearly all wards, there are certain rules which have to be obeyed. Things are much less starchy than they used to be, but even today you will be asked to conform to regulations and timetables which may not be entirely to your taste.

None the less, a hernia operation is only going to keep you in hospital for a few days, so you shouldn't find it too difficult to fall in with ward routine during that time.

Mixed wards

Mixed wards (in which there are both men and women patients) seem to be a peculiarly British invention. They were introduced during the 1970s – with, as far as I know, absolutely no consultation with the patients – as a way of saving money.

Over the years, it has become more and more apparent that many people distrust them. In particular, a lot of women deeply dislike the idea of having unknown males tucked up in the next bed.

It seems likely that many mixed wards are going to be phased out, simply because of the public's distaste for them. The hospital should tell you, well before you are admitted, whether there is any likelihood of your going into a mixed ward. If you don't fancy the idea, say so: alternative arrangements should then be made for you.

The staff

Just a brief word about the medical staff whom you'll meet while you're in the ward having your hernia operation.

The doctors

In an NHS ward, there's quite a rigid, hierarchical structure, which looks something like this:

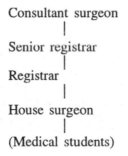

Consultant surgeon
|
Senior registrar
|
Registrar
|
House surgeon
|
(Medical students)

Obviously, it's a pecking order. The consultant surgeon is the boss, and very much so. He (nearly all hernia surgeons are men, I'm afraid) is a highly qualified and experienced person, aged between about 38 and 65. The team he leads is usually called 'a firm'. The next person down the chain of command is likely to be the senior registrar, and below her is often a registrar. These are both well-qualified and skilful surgeons.

Working for them is the house surgeon. He is a recently qualified doctor, working on a six-month contract. Much of the donkey work of the firm is done by this hard-pressed (and often exhausted) individual.

Finally, in teaching hospitals (and some other large hospitals which have links with them), there will be some medical students attached to the firm. They're mainly there to be taught by the qualified staff, but they also do some of the practical work, like taking blood and (maybe) assisting at your operation. When you're first admitted, they may well come and take down your medical history, and examine you.

If you don't want to be examined by medical students, you can say so. But most patients like being seen by them – and sometimes they do actually discover important things which have been missed by their more senior colleagues!

In a private hospital, the system is far simpler. The surgeon comes in to see you and to do your operation, and that's about it. He does not have junior staff to help him – though there may be a duty medical officer who is available in case of emergencies.

Incidentally, one doctor who is missing from the above list is your *anaesthetist*. She isn't part of the firm, and instead works in a separate anaesthesia department (there is more about the anaesthetist in the section on general anaesthesia below).

The nurses

Whether you're in a private or an NHS hospital, you'll be looked after by a highly trained and very caring team of nurses. If you have worries about your hernia operation, don't hesitate to chat to one of them and ask her advice.

In the NHS these days, there's often a system whereby you have a 'named nurse' to look after you. She is familiar with your case, and will try and help you with any queries you may have.

Naturally, there are many other ward staff. Nowadays most people wear name-badges which indicate what their job is.

Preparation for the operation

On the morning of your operation, several things will happen:

• You won't be given any breakfast. In fact, the nurses should hang a sign on your bed saying 'Nil by mouth'. This is because you're going to have a general anaesthetic. Regrettably, mistakes can occur on busy wards – so if somebody comes along and offers you any food or drink, you must refuse it.

- You'll be shaved round the area of the rupture; the staff may give you a razor and invite you to do this yourself.
- You'll be asked to sign a consent form (see below).
- You'll be given pre-medication (a 'pre-med'). This drug is designed to make the operation easier, and to relax you. It may be given as an injection or in tablet-form.

The consent form

As you'll know if you have read the earlier part of this chapter (on day-case surgery), the surgeon will not be willing to operate on your hernia until you have signed a consent form.

The consent form varies a little from hospital to hospital, but basically it's a legal document which says that you agree to the hernia operation – and that you understand what is going to be done to you.

Do not sign the form unless you really do understand what is going to happen. If you are not clear, ask a doctor to explain it to you in more understandable terms.

SAMPLE CONSENT FORM FOR HERNIA OPERATION

<u>ST ELSEWHERE'S HOSPITAL</u>
<u>CONSENT FOR OPERATION</u>

I, __WILLIAM JONES__ , of 1 HIGH ST, ANYTOWN, hereby consent to the operation of __HERNIA REPAIR__ , the nature and effects of which have been explained to me by the doctor named below.

I also consent to such further measures as might be found necessary during the operation.

No assurance has been given to me that the operation will be performed by a particular surgeon.

Signed _____ Date _____

I confirm that I have explained the nature of the operation and the type of anaesthetic to the patient in terms which he has understood.

Name (Dr) __B. TROVATO__
Signed _____

In an NHS hospital, the consent form will specify that you have not been told that one particular doctor will do the operation. This means that the consultant surgeon is free to delegate the hernia repair to one of his juniors if he so chooses.

There's one other aspect of the hernia operation consent form of which male patients must be aware. Very occasionally – and especially in older men – the hole through which the hernia has passed is so big and so difficult to repair that the surgeon feels he has to remove the testicle. There are more details about this procedure in Chapter 9. But if you are worried about this possibility, do not sign the consent form until you have talked matters over with one of the surgical team.

Some consent forms specifically say, 'I have told the doctor about any additional procedures which I do not wish to be carried out.' However, merely telling someone that you do not want your testicle removed might be of limited legal value. If you feel strongly about this, it would be best if you write on the consent form, by hand, the words, 'No removal of testicle, please.'

General anaesthetic

The doctor who visits you in the ward to explain the operation and get the consent form signed should also tell you anything you want to know about the general anaesthetic.

You may also get a pre-operation visit from the anaesthetist, particularly if you are in a private hospital.

Incidentally, anaesthetists tell me that some patients don't know who they are, don't realize that they are doctors, and think that they are technicians or porters! In fact, an anaesthetist (called an 'anesthesiologist' in the USA and some other countries) is a very highly skilled physician who is expert in putting people to sleep, keeping them safe during the operation – and waking them up again afterwards.

You've almost certainly heard that very rarely an anaesthetic goes badly wrong, and someone dies or is brain-damaged. The chances of this happening during a hernia operation, with a competent anaesthetist at a good hospital, are very remote indeed.

By the time the anaesthetist gets to work on you, you may well be a little drowsy from the pre-med. (The drugs may also have made your mouth a little dry.) She normally anaesthetizes you in a special room next to the operating theatre – but sometimes you may be wheeled straight into theatre and anaesthetized there.

Almost certainly, what will happen is that the anaesthetist will put a needle into a vein in your hand or arm (this is almost painless) and inject a sleep-inducing drug. Within about 10 seconds this will reach your brain, and out you go. The next thing you know, you'll be waking up in your bed – and the hernia operation will be over.

After the operation

You're bound to feel rather woozy and tired for the first couple of hours after coming round, so just take things easy and relax. Don't attempt to do anything for yourself till you're completely together.

The likelihood is that you will feel little pain from the site of the rupture operation. This is because:

* The drugs given to you while you were anaesthetized are still giving you protection against pain;
* The anaesthetist may have put a pain-relieving suppository in your back passage – a lot of British people do not like this, so it is often the practice to ask your permission before the operation;
* Even though you have had a general anaesthetic, the surgeon may well have injected a long-acting local anaesthetic around the operation site. This may make you a little unsteady on your feet when you start walking.

When and if you do feel any significant pain, ask the nurses for a tablet to ease it.

Curiously enough, some people feel practically no pain at all in the hours which follow the operation. Others feel a moderate amount – especially when they cough or laugh. There's currently a theory that the older you are, the less pain you feel.

Getting mobile

There's no doubt that the sooner you can get mobile after a hernia operation (or any other surgical procedure), the better it is for your health. Getting up and about reduces your chances of thrombosis (blood clotting) and of chest infection.

These days some surgeons may actually want you to walk a few steps on the evening after your operation – and on the following day you will certainly be asked to move around the ward without overdoing things. You may find it helpful to put your hand over the operation site when you're moving – both to support it and protect it.

Going to the loo

Because you've had an operation – and been 'starved' for a short period – you may not have a bowel action for a day or two; this does not matter. It is a waste of time to take laxatives.

As far as passing urine is concerned, you should have done this within about eight hours of coming round. If you haven't, then tell a nurse. In older men, prostate trouble can start playing up immediately after a hernia operation, and it's important to spot that this is happening.

The incision site

A cut several inches long has been made in your groin (as shown in Figure 7). It has been stitched up, or possibly clipped with metal staples – in fact, these days there may be *no* stitching visible, as the surgeon may have done it all just below the skin.

You'll probably have some form of gauze dressing over the cut. It's quite likely that the nurses will replace this with a spray-on dressing of 'plastic skin'. This keeps things clean, while letting the staff see how you're healing up.

Going home

Most people think that there is some officially laid-down period of time which you must spend in hospital after a rupture operation. This simply isn't true: it depends entirely on the surgeon who is in charge of your case, and what his preferences are. About 25 years ago, Dr David Owen, (the same David Owen who became Foreign Secretary and is now Lord Owen) did a most valuable piece of research in which he found that some surgeons kept patients in for 12 days – while others turned them out in two! There was no rhyme or reason to this.

Under today's pressures to get patients out of hospital quickly, the average hernia stay is very much shorter. Some surgeons may keep you in for two days – others for three or four. (And day-case surgery is very much a possibility, as described earlier in this chapter.)

Of course, if you're not very well – for instance, if you get a post-operative chest infection – you might have to stay in a few days longer.

The doctors should be able to forecast your discharge date, so that you can make appropriate arrangements to go home. You shouldn't drive yourself, just in case you don't have proper control of your legs yet – nor should you use public transport. For a little while, you need a bit of mollycoddling – as we shall see in the next chapter.

7

Coping at home after the operation

The operation is over, and you're out of hospital. How are you going to cope over the next few weeks?

Much depends on which type of operation you've had. In general, recovery from the new day-case operations is a good deal quicker than recovery from the traditional type of hernia repair. But remember that people vary greatly. During your recovery, be guided by what your surgeon has told you about how soon you should do things – but do not let yourself get tired out.

Getting home

When you get home, you probably will be quite weary – especially if you've been an in-patient in hospital and have had a general anaesthetic.

So make a resolution that you're going to take life easy for the next few days. If you have a partner or relatives living with you, then let them take the strain for a day or two. It should be up to them to bring you meals and do the shopping. If you live on your own, then just try and do as little as possible for at least 72 hours. (A good plan is to lay in some shopping before you go into hospital.)

The next few weeks

Over the next few weeks, you'll be able to increase the pace of your activities quite markedly – especially if you have had an open mesh operation or keyhole surgery.

If there are any stitches to come out, this will probably be done about a week or so after the operation, either by the hospital or by your GP. By that time, the incision will probably have healed up very well, though it may stick up a little bit from the surface of your skin. This is nothing to worry about (but see the note below about infection). A little bruising around and below the wound is normal; it will go away soon.

Will there be much pain?

After the first couple of days, there should be very little pain in your groin, though for a little while you may feel like protecting it slightly with your hand when you move around.

Painkilling tablets can usually be stopped about five days after the operation. If you feel that pain is persisting for an abnormally long time, check with your doctor.

Will there be bleeding?

Slight blood loss on the dressing during the first day or two is normal; after that it should go away.

Heavy bleeding is most unlikely. If it occurs, press a pad very firmly on your groin, and either ring your GP or else go to the nearest hospital with an Accident & Emergency department.

Looking out for infection

Any surgical incision can become infected, though the odds are against this happening with a simple rupture operation. But if the area of the cut suddenly gets tender or becomes red (or unusually dark if you're of African or Asian ancestry), then get medical advice within a couple of hours. Another likely sign of infection is yellow pus exuding from the hernia incision.

Fortunately, the great majority of infections which occur after this type of operation are easily dealt with. The doctors will usually take a swab to send to the lab for testing (to see which germs are present) and then put you on antibiotics.

'Crusting' along the line of the cut is not a sign of infection. Crusts usually develop about a week after the operation, and gradually fall off.

Odd feelings round the cut

You may have odd feelings round the cut, such as tingling and numbness. This is quite normal, and is just due to the fact that inevitably some small nerve-endings have to be cut through during the operation.

These odd feelings will gradually get less, but can persist for quite a few months.

How much can I walk?

After the first day or so at home, you can walk as much as you like. (Remember that in the first 24 hours after the actual operation, your leg may be a bit wobbly because of local anaesthetic which has been injected into your groin.)

I'm not suggesting that you go mountain-walking the morning after you get home, but the exercise of a stroll will be good for you. A possible programme for getting fit again would be:

First day after return home: Walk 200 metres (about 200 yards).
Second day: Walk 400 metres (about 400 yards).
Third day: Walk 800 metres (about half a mile).
Fourth day: Walk 1.5 km (about a mile).
Fifth day and subsequently: try and walk at least 1.5 km a day (a mile) – or get some other equivalent exercise.

If you're not very keen on walking, a good alternative is swimming, which you should be able to do as soon as the wound has dried up.

What can I do around the house?
Work around the house – whether it's cleaning, doing repairs or whatever – does tend to involve a lot of bending and stretching. This is not a good idea in the early days after a hernia repair, since there is a chance that you could dislodge internal stitches and perhaps lead to a recurrence of the rupture (see below).

So: DIY tasks, polishing the floor, getting things off top shelves, climbing into the attic, shifting the furniture, and so on – all of these should be *out* during the first few weeks after you come home.

The same applies to gardening, except for the very gentle, pottering kind.

Eating
Once you get home you can eat what you like – though on the first night after day-case surgery, you should stick to a light meal.

Having a diet which is rich in fibre will help to keep your bowels regular, and will assist you in keeping your weight down. This lessens the chance of a recurrence of your hernia.

Fibre-containing foods include cereals, wholemeal bread, fruit and vegetables.

Foods to avoid if you want to keep your weight down are those which contain fat. It's not an exaggeration to say that tucking into too much fat could eventually make your hernia recur.

Bathing and washing

Unless your surgeon tells you differently, you can have a bath or shower about five days after your rupture operation. If there is any wound-dressing (such as gauze) you'll probably have been told that you can remove it at this stage. After that, just keep the operation site clean; a gentle wash each day is fine, without a lot of hard rubbing.

After a wash or bath, dry the area gently and thoroughly. A little talcum powder shaken over the groin is fine, because it helps to avoid uncomfortable friction between your skin and your clothes.

Talc also helps ease the slight discomfort caused by stubbly hair regrowing around the operation zone.

Lifting

If you're in any doubt about lifting anything during the weeks after your rupture operation – *don't*. As we've seen, lifting increases the pressure inside your abdomen. Therefore, it can increase the chances of your hernia recurring.

Lifting very trivial weights (for instance, picking up a pair of shoes or a teapot) is totally harmless. But you must use your common sense about even the most moderate weights.

And as for anything heavy: forget it. Personally, I wouldn't even lift a two-year-old toddler during the first month or so after a hernia operation.

How soon can I drive?

Most surgeons wouldn't be too keen on you starting driving within 10 days of surgery.

As described above, local anaesthetic injected into the operation site could make your leg difficult to control immediately after the operation. And even after that wears off, your groin will be stiff. You might not be able to operate the pedals easily – particularly in an emergency.

Warning: your car insurance company might not cover you if you drove too soon after your operation. So be guided by your surgeon.

How soon can I make love?

Contrary to what some folk imagine, most people who undergo hernia surgery are still interested in sex. Fortunately, you can resume making love as soon as you wish. As would be the case after any operation, you should avoid sudden and violent movements – in order to avoid 'pulling' stitches – during the first few weeks.

There's a great deal of misunderstanding about the relationship between hernias and sexual activity: more about this in Chapter 9.

How soon can I go back to work?

How soon you return to work after a hernia operation depends on:

- the nature of your work;
- the type of operation you've had (traditional, keyhole or mesh).

After the traditional operation, a desk-bound person might reasonably expect to be back in his office chair within three weeks. But the same person might well manage to resume working only a few days after keyhole or mesh surgery. However, he would have to be guided by his surgeon. (And when you're sitting at your desk, don't get any ideas about lifting word-processors around the office!)

The situation is very different for anyone who does heavy work – especially work involving lifting. After a traditional-style hernia operation, excessive strain could cause recurrence of the hernia. The Royal College of Surgeons says that 'heavy work such as labouring' may be resumed one month after a traditional type of operation – but your own surgeon may not necessarily feel that this is a good idea. After the open mesh operation or after keyhole surgery, most surgeons will let you resume reasonably heavy work within a fortnight.

However, if you have the slightest pain during any activity, the safest rule is to stop. You don't want a recurrence (see below).

Recurrence

Recurrence means that the hernia comes back, and starts bulging through your groin again. Happily, this is not likely to occur during the first few weeks after you go home. However, if by chance you notice that your groin is developing a lump again, do go to your GP for a check-up. This is not actually an emergency, since no immediate action can be taken to put it right. However, you should keep your feet up as much as possible until you can see your GP.

In practice, recurrence – which is much commoner than most people realize – isn't likely to happen for some months or years after the operation. Your best chances of preventing it lie in:

- keeping your weight down;
- getting a reasonable amount of exercise;
- avoiding heavy lifting and excessive physical stresses;
- avoiding repeated coughing;
- avoiding straining on the toilet.

It's well worth trying to follow the above rules. Sadly, a recurrent hernia is not always curable by having a repeat operation – that's why many people who have a recurrence end up having to wear a truss (see Chapter 8).

8

Trusses and other non-surgical strategies

We've seen that the best treatment for a hernia is to have it repaired, by an operation. But are there any alternatives?

Yes: you can survive – and *perhaps* lead a reasonably active life – without surgery. Indeed, if you're one of the tiny minority of people who are totally unfit for an operation, then obviously you have to look at the only other reasonably successful way of controlling your rupture – the use of a truss.

What is a truss – and who needs one?

A truss is a sort of belt. A typical one is shown in Figure 8. You can see that there's a pad about the size of a small egg at one end of it. The idea is that the pad is worn directly over the hole in your groin, so that it keeps the hernia from coming out.

These days, most trusses are made of elastic material, so that quite a bit of pressure is exerted on the pad. Usually there are one or two

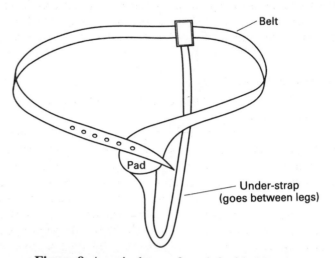

Figure 8 A typical truss for a left-sided hernia.

straps to hold it in place, which pass back between the patient's legs and fasten on to the belt somewhere above his bottom.

Double trusses, which have two pads instead of one, are made for the small group of people who are unlucky enough to have a hernia on both sides of the body (called a double rupture).

Some firms now produce neat, trunks-style trusses (see Figure 9), in which the pad is actually built into the front of what appears at first sight to be rather bulky jockey-type underpants.

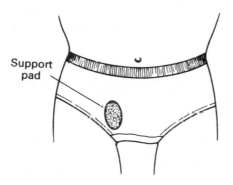

Figure 9 A trunks-style truss.

There's also an older type of truss called a 'spring band', which has no understraps. It contains a strong steel spring which exerts pressure on the pad. It's much less common than the modern elastic type.

A warning about trusses

Trusses can be dangerous. Do not get one unless a surgeon has advised you to do so.

Why are they dangerous? First of all, one type of rupture (a femoral hernia – see Chapter 3) simply cannot be controlled by a truss. And this particular kind of hernia is especially liable to serious complications, such as strangulation. Therefore, if you have a femoral hernia, you are simply inviting disaster by wearing a truss.

Furthermore, a truss may actually cause problems for people who suffer from *any* kind of hernia. This is because the devices exert considerable pressure – and if the pressure is on slightly the wrong area, the result may be a strangulated hernia (see Chapter 4).

There are two circumstances in which a truss could cause this kind of trouble:

- if the patient hasn't put it on properly;
- if the patient hasn't been measured and fitted for it correctly in the first place.

Later in this chapter, you'll find advice about where to get a truss fitted – and about how to put it on.

Who needs trusses?

In an ideal world, everyone who has a rupture would have it cured by hernia surgery, and then no one would need a truss. However, life is more complicated than that, and the following groups of people often end up wearing these supports:

- Those who are scared stiff of surgery, and cannot bring themselves to go 'under the knife'.
- Those who are too ill to undergo surgery. This mainly means elderly people with very bad heart or lung problems. However, these days some surgeons feel that almost anyone can safely have one of the new operations (such as the open mesh technique) under local anaesthetic.
- Those who have very small hernias of the type known as direct inguinal (a term which is explained in Chapter 3). Direct inguinal hernias are different from other types of ruptures, in that they seldom cause serious problems. So there is sometimes a case for just controlling them with a truss.
- Many people who have recurrent hernias (see Chapter 7) are not really suitable for a second operation, and are therefore given trusses.

Where to get a truss

You'll have gathered from the above that you need to be carefully fitted for a truss. Buying one which doesn't fit your body is idiotic – it's rather like getting size five shoes when you have size nine feet.

So who does the fitting? The most skilled people at this particular business are called orthotists, though in some parts of the world they are still referred to as truss-fitters.

Fully trained orthotists are available at most of the large general hospitals in the UK. Normally, you get to see them through being referred by a surgeon, who has decided that your rupture is suitable for a truss. However, in the last year or two, some British hospitals have been willing to fit trusses on patients who have been sent by fund-holding GPs (i.e. patients who haven't seen a surgeon). Whether this trend will continue is uncertain.

The orthotist works in a hospital department which is either called Orthotics or, more simply, Surgical Appliances. Before your visit he will have had a letter from the surgeon, explaining exactly which type of hernia you have. He'll take you into a private room, ask you to strip off, and then take various measurements of your body – a procedure which doesn't take very long.

Having got your statistics, he will take a suitable truss from his stocks and put it on you. As explained above, the belt goes round you, just below the waist, with a couple of thin straps probably passing backwards between your thighs. The pad itself rests over your groin. If you're a man, and you have the type of inguinal hernia that runs down into the scrotum, then your truss probably has a rather longer pad which comes down toward the scrotal area.

The orthotist will make sure that you're really comfortable in the truss, and will get you to cough and to move about in it. Then he will check that you yourself can put the truss on without difficulty – the most important thing being that you should be able to push the hernia back into your body before applying the pad to the site.

The whole process of fitting a truss, and teaching you how to put it on and take it off, doesn't usually take more than 15 minutes. At the end of it, you will be the proud owner of your own personal truss – and at an NHS hospital, you won't have to pay anything for it.

Don't hesitate to ring or go back to the orthotist if the truss is ever uncomfortable, or if you're having any problems with it. You'll probably have to go back and see him at some stage in any case, because the device may wear out after a while.

It's not generally realized (even by doctors) that trusses don't last for ever. A young, active man may wear one out quite quickly – perhaps in six to 12 monhs. So if your truss starts to 'give', and doesn't seem to be providing you with proper support, contact the orthotist.

Getting trusses from chemists

Some people prefer to obtain their trusses privately (rather than on the NHS), via a pharmacy. There are one or two very large pharmacies – particularly in the West End of London – where a professional truss-fitter comes in and does sessions. However, if you decide to buy one through your local chemist, then it will probably be the branch manager who invites you into a back room and takes your measurements.

My opinion is that the shop manager – no matter how well-meaning she may be – will probably not have a vast experience in fitting trusses. On the other hand, it's quite a cheap way of buying: in Britain at the present time, the cost of a truss obtained through a chemist's tends to be between £29 and £50, depending on which type of device you choose. This is certainly a good deal less than you would pay if you went to a hospital privately; hospital charges tend to be about double the above – though you are paying for the skill and experience of the orthotist.

Ordering trusses by post

Each year, tens of thousands of people buy mail-order trusses from the firms who advertise in newspapers. Again, the costs tend to be low – £25 to £45 at present in Britain.

But the obvious problem is that the person who supplies the truss never sees you. The following things could therefore go wrong:

- Unknown to the suppliers, you might have a femoral hernia – the type that cannot be controlled by trusses.
- The truss might not fit you properly.
- Because there's no one to help you, you might be putting it on incorrectly and perhaps causing yourself harm.

Having said all that, there's probably quite a good case for getting *replacement* trusses by mail if you want to – as long as you were properly measured and fitted by an expert in the first place.

Using trusses properly

It's quite easy to use a truss the wrong way, and thus cause yourself problems. Reputable manufacturers issue guidelines similar to these:

1 Push your hernia back into your body before putting on the truss.

2 Wear the truss next to your skin – *not* over your undergarments.
3 Keep it tight enough to hold the rupture in place at all times.
4 Put the truss on when you get up in the morning, and if possible wear it all day.
5 Unless you have been told otherwise by your surgeon or orthotist, remove the truss when you go to bed.
6 Keep your skin clean, and the truss clean.
7 If your skin chafes under the pressure of the truss, apply lots of talcum powder. Some people put alcohol on the skin, but this should be kept away from the truss, as it may harm it.
8 If the truss is uncomfortable, see your orthotist or doctor.
9 If you have any pain, then there may be something medically wrong. Check with your doctor right away (see below).

Pain and trusses

If you've read the early part of this book, you'll know that the big danger with a hernia is the risk of complications – and particularly strangulation (which occurs when the blood supply to the lump is cut off).

Truss-wearers are liable to complications, simply because their hernias have not been cured. It is particularly important that truss-users are always on the look-out for strangulation – which, after all, can readily kill you if it is not detected promptly.

So if you get actual pain in your hernia, don't ignore it! Go and lie down, take off the truss, and see if the pain goes away.

If it hasn't gone within half an hour, *ring your doctor*. If he thinks that there is the slightest chance of strangulation, he will examine you as soon as possible.

Other devices and methods

Apart from trusses, there are some other devices which can help control hernias in the groin and elsewhere. These include abdominal supports – which are rather like corsets – and special bags for large scrotal hernias. There are also now some very lightweight 'hernia aids', which are small groin supports used for sporting activities and even swimming.

Some of these devices can be bought by mail order – though you should check with your surgeon before wearing one which you've acquired in this way. Others are supplied by hospitals. And in certain cases, your hospital's Orthotics Department may have to make a specially designed support for you in their workshop.

Postural relief of hernias

If it's been decided that your rupture can't be operated on, it's worth your while remembering that, *for short periods only*, it's possible to keep the lump under control by postural means. In other words, if you're having a difficult day, go and lie down! Use your fingers to push the bulge back through the hole in your groin. And stay lying down till you feel better.

This postural technique works even better if the foot of your bed has been raised slightly.

Note: if you get any pain, contact your GP (see above).

Alternative remedies

Rupture is one field of medicine where alternative (complementary) practitioners can do nothing. But for the sake of completeness I ought to say that some of them *claim* to be able to help.

For example, certain homeopathic and naturopathic textbooks say that Nux Vomica (a well-known traditional medication) is 'a good remedy for hernia'. Without wishing to be unfair to complementary practitioners, I must say that if you happen to have a hole the size of a golf ball in your groin, it's a little difficult to see how any medicine could mysteriously make it disappear.

Similarly, some reflexology books maintain that certain pressures on the sole of the foot are good for ruptures. Again, I must stress that I know of nothing on earth (other than surgery) which will make a hole in the groin heal up.

Some alternative treatments may make you *feel* better while you're suffering from a hernia – but they can't make it go away.

Summary

Summing up this chapter, it's clear that the best way of dealing with a hernia is to have it cured by an operation. But if that's not possible, then a truss (or similar device) could well help. However, make sure that it's well-fitted, and that you use it correctly.

9

Groin hernias and sex

A lot of hernia patients are secretly worried that the condition – or the operation – will affect their sex lives.

This isn't surprising. After all, a groin rupture is very close to your sex organs; indeed, in men the bulge may actually come down into the scrotum so that it lies next to the testicle. Furthermore, many people have heard jokes – particularly when they were youngsters – about hernias 'ruining your married life'. Several of my school-friends believed that lifting a weight with your legs apart would 'rupture your testicles'.

A further complication is that until recent years, many doctors – and virtually all hernia surgeons – totally ignored the question of sexual function when talking to their patients. That really shouldn't happen today.

Does a hernia interfere with your sex life?

Will a hernia interfere with your sex life? The short answer is 'No'. There's no reason why the mere fact of having a small gap in your abdominal wall should spoil your love life, whether you're male or female. There's no real connection between the hernia and your reproductive apparatus.

Having said that, I must add that to have a bulge so near to your genitals isn't really conducive to enjoying a rampaging sex life with your partner, especially if the lump is uncomfortable or causing you pain. Indeed, in recent years one or two people who have sued their employers, because of ruptures which were allegedly caused by work, have also claimed that their hernias provoked pain in the genitals and interfered with sexual function. It is not clear whether the courts accepted these claims.

Does the operation interfere with your sex life?

Will the operation itself harm your sex life? That's a secret fear which haunts quite a lot of people – especially men!

Be reassured: literally thousands of people undergo hernia surgery each month, and it is very rare for any of them to complain of sexual problems afterwards. None the less, after *any* operation (no matter what it is), it occasionally happens that the person runs into sexual problems, such as impotence. The cause for this is not clear, since often there is no physical reason why an operation should cause this kind of difficulty. It may be that the sheer stress of undergoing an operation is to blame.

But a hernia repair is not usually a very stressful operation – especially when you have it done as a day case. Most people stroll through it, and resume their sex lives afterwards without any difficulty. Over my long medical career – which has involved receiving tens of thousands of letters from all over the world about sexual problems – I cannot recall any patients who have complained that rupture surgery caused them impotence, or any other sexual difficulty.

Nevertheless, there are a few facts of which you ought to be aware:

- In the unlikely event that a hernia operation (or any operation in that part of the body, for that matter) goes wrong, there will probably be pain. And pain itself limits sexual function. For instance, in the wildly unlikely event that you got a serious groin infection as a result of a rupture operation, then the resultant discomfort and aching might well put paid to sexual intercourse for a while.
- People who sue their employers over ruptures caused by heavy work do sometimes complain that pain and numbness are present in the genitals after surgery. One man claimed that his testicle had got smaller, but it is not clear whether the court accepted this.
- Most importantly, in older male patients it is occasionally necessary to remove the testicle during hernia surgery.

Removal of a testicle during surgery

Why might a testicle have to be removed? Unfortunately, the hole through which the hernia has bulged is sometimes so big that it is very difficult to repair. And the spermatic cord – which is the testicle's lifeline, and carries its blood supply – runs right through the hole. The surgeon may feel that he simply cannot close up the gap without cutting through the spermatic cord – an action which means losing the testicle.

72

It's fortunate that this testicle-removal is rarely necessary except in very old men, whose sex lives are likely to be less active. In any case, a man can usually have one testicle removed and continue to function adequately with the other one.

I must stress very strongly: *if there is any risk that testicle-removal might become necessary, the surgeon should discuss this with you beforehand and get your permission.*

In days gone by, this permission was often not obtained, and the procedure was simply carried out – especially on older patients. The implication was that OAPs don't have sex – something which we now know to be totally untrue. These days, surgeons are much better about appreciating that their patients may actually have sex lives. But if you're an older man and are at all worried that your testicle might be removed during rupture surgery, then make sure that you talk things over with the surgeon or one of his team well beforehand.

And (as suggested in Chapter 6) do not sign a consent form which would give your surgeon *carte blanche* to take away your testicle without your permission.

Summary

In case you have been alarmed by reading any of the last few pages, let me repeat that in the vast majority of cases, hernia surgery will not have the slightest effect on your sex life. According to the Royal College of Surgeon's advice on the subject, you may resume sexual intercourse as soon as your groin feels comfortable enough.

Incidentally, the College asks patients to note that a hernia repair is *not* a sterilization operation! So it certainly won't stop you having children.

10

Hernias in children

If you're a patient who's been told that your child has a hernia, you probably haven't bothered to plough through the early chapters of this book, which explain about adult hernias. So let me recap on a few basic facts.

- 'Hernia' and 'rupture' mean exactly the same thing.
- A hernia is a bulge which has pushed its way through a gap in the body.
- The gap is usually a congenital weak point (i.e. something you're born with).
- The bulge often consists of intestine ('gut'), but may have other structures in it.

An important fact for you, as a parent, to grasp is that the hernia is *not* your fault (or anybody else's fault either). Hernias in children are common. They are not due to anything the mother did (like smoking, drinking or taking medication) during pregnancy. As far as we know, they just happen. So don't blame yourself – or the doctors or nurses.

Fortunately, the average childhood rupture is fairly straightforward. If surgery is necessary, it should provide a rapid and straightforward cure. And surgery may well not be necessary: children are different from adults in that some hernias – the ones which occur at the navel – will often cure themselves.

We'll begin by discussing groin hernias, move on to navel (umbilical) hernias, and then deal with one or two much rarer types of childhood hernia.

Groin hernias in childhood

Hernias tend to be associated in people's minds with middle and old age, so parents are usually very surprised to be told that their baby has a rupture. Yet the truth is that groin hernias are very common in childhood: no fewer than one in 50 of all boy babies has one. Girls don't get them so frequently, but one in every few hundred female babies develops a hernia. Indeed, the curing of groin hernias is actually the commonest of all forms of paediatric surgery.

Why are these little bulges so prone to occur? As explained in Chapter 2, the groin is a distinctly weak area of the body in both sexes – and more particularly so in males, because of their testicles. Testicles start off *inside* the human body, but during the seventh month of pregnancy, they actually travel out of the baby's abdomen and go down into his scrotum. In order to do this, they have to pass through a tiny gap in the groin. (There's a similar gap in girls, but it's not so big.)

When the testicle reaches the scrotum, everything should close up behind it. But in many boys, this just doesn't happen. Instead, the child is left with a little sac (like the finger of a rubber glove) which goes through the gap in his groin, and down towards his scrotum (see Figure 10). So it's now very easy for structures in his abdomen – such as a piece of intestine – to push into that sac and cause a bulge in his groin.

And that's when you notice that something is wrong . . .

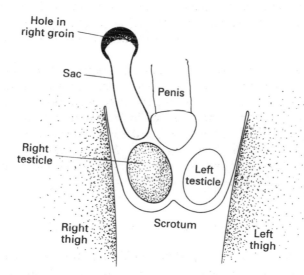

Figure 10 Congenital sac which increases the risk of a childhood groin hernia.

What do you notice?

How do you know that your baby's got a hernia? The main symptom is a bulging in the groin. Most commonly, it's the father or mother who first spots it, rather than a doctor. Often, you're changing a nappy and you suddenly observe that there's some sort of a lump, located two or three centimetres (an inch or so) to one side of the genitals.

Very frequently, the bulge is only obvious when the child is crying – since that increases the pressure inside the abdomen (belly), and pushes the hernia outwards. At other times, when the baby is quiet, there may well be no lump at all.

How old is the child likely to be when the swelling is discovered? In boys, it's usually spotted when they're very young: the great majority are under a year old, and many are less than three months. In girls, however, the lump may not appear till quite a bit later – often not till they're several years old.

Incidentally, not *all* groin lumps in children are due to hernias. So if you find a swelling in your youngster's groin, it could be due to other things, such as:

- an undescended testicle;
- a hydrocoele (pronounced HIDE-ro-seal), which is a collection of fluid;
- an enlarged gland.

What to do

If you discover a lump in your child's groin, there's no need to panic. Unless he is in pain, this isn't an emergency. However, you should make an appointment to see your GP within the next two or three days. In the meantime, you needn't do anything in particular, like change the child's diet or restrict his activities.

Fortunately, most children who have hernias are so very young that they're completely unaware that anything is wrong with them. As they can't even talk, you don't have to worry about discussing the swelling with them. But if you're in the unusual situation of finding a possible hernia in a child who *is* old enough to talk and to understand, take care not to make a big deal of the matter. Reassure the child that the little bump is nothing to worry about, and that the doctor will take a look at it in a day or two.

Warning: if a lump is painful, you must ring up your GP and insist on being seen within an hour or two. This is because of the risk of the complication called strangulation (see below). If for any reason your doctor is unavailable, take the child to the nearest hospital Accident & Emergency department.

Treatment

There is only one treatment for a groin hernia in childhood, and that is to operate on it. Don't let anybody convince you otherwise. Folk remedies and wait-and-see tactics will not work.

Furthermore, a childhood groin rupture has to be operated on *soon*, and not just left for months and months. This is because of the risk that strangulation might occur. In strangulation, the blood supply to the hernia gets cut off. This causes pain – and gangrene can develop very rapidly. So you can see that it's a very serious business.

That's why your child needs to have his groin hernia cured as rapidly as possible. Your GP will examine him, confirm the diagnosis of a rupture – and then arrange for him to be seen by a surgeon. In an ideal world, this should be within a week or two.

It is best if your youngster sees a paediatric surgeon – who is constantly dealing with childhood hernias. However, there are some parts of the world where this is just not possible, so you may have to take the baby to a general surgeon.

At the present time, I would strongly advise against taking your child to one of the new and widely publicized hernia clinics. These are geared to dealing with adult types of rupture, and they're fine for that. But babies need to be dealt with by people whose speciality is babies.

The operation

The surgeon will get your child into hospital as soon as is reasonably possible. The only real reason for delay would be if the youngster had a bad cold or a chest infection.

Surgery is normally performed under general anaesthetic, so your child won't feel a thing. The 'pre-med' may well put her to sleep before she even goes to the operating theatre.

The surgeon makes a small cut – usually about 2.5 cms (an inch) or so long – in the fold of the groin, just where the belly meets the thigh. Once under the skin, he finds the little sac (pouch) of the rupture, and simply removes it. Then he stitches up – and that's it. This operation is called a herniotomy – a medical word meaning 'removal of a hernia'. It is *not* the same as the common adult operation of herniorrhaphy, which involves heavy darning.

One thing you should know beforehand is that a child who has a rupture on one side often turns out to have one on the other side too. Therefore, it's highly probable that the paediatric surgeon will make a small incision in the other groin, to see if that too has a hernia sac that needs removing.

Your baby should have very little post-operative pain, and should be able to take feeds within a very short time.

Provided there are no complicating factors, he should be out of hospital within a couple of days, and be completely back to normal almost immediately. The surgical staff will advise you whether any stitches need removing, and will tell you what to do about dressings.

You needn't take any particular precautions, except to ensure for a week or two that he doesn't bang himself in the groin area.

Recurrence

Though adult groin hernias very frequently recur (in other words, break through again), this is extremely rare in childhood. So once your youngster has had his groin rupture removed, both you and he can forget all about it.

Psychological aspects of groin hernias

You have to bear in mind that this operation is in an area very close to the child's genitals. Is this likely to cause any psychological effects?

In most cases, the answer is 'No'. As we've seen, most boys have their rupture operations when they're far too small to know anything about it.

But some children – including a high proportion of the relatively small number of girls who have hernias – do have the operation when they're quite a bit older. In these cases, it's very important to reassure the youngster that:

- the operation is perfectly safe;
- there won't be a lot of pain;
- it won't harm their sexual parts.

Older children – and indeed their parents – may be pleased to know that an uncomplicated hernia operation will not affect sexual function, nor the chances of having a family.

Finally, a note about the scar: any child who has a groin hernia operated on will bear a small scar for the rest of his life. But it is usually a very thin one, disguised by the fold of the groin, and likely to be hidden later on by the pubic hair. It's very unlikely that other people will notice it. When the child himself spots it, it's sensible to tell him openly that he had a small and trivial lump there as a baby – but that surgeons were able to remove it.

Umbilical (navel) hernias in children

The navel is one of the weak points of the body. This is simply because it's the spot where the umbilical cord passed through the wall of the abdomen – so there's a potential gap there. Any potential gap in the human body may turn into a hernia; in other words, something may bulge through it. Therefore, it's not surprising that navel hernias are very common indeed.

In fact, some experts say that as many as *one in five* of all new-born babies have a small hernia here. However, this may be an exaggeration – most of these tiny bulges are never noticed by anyone, and simply go away during the first few weeks of life.

But in a lot of children, there is a more definite hernia: a bulge located at the navel which is sufficiently prominent to be noted by a parent, doctor or nurse. Typically, the bulge comes up when the baby cries or struggles or strains to pass a motion. The swelling feels rather tense. You can push it back into the belly with your finger-tips, and it may well go back with an audible gurgle; this is because it contains a little piece of bowel (gut or intestine).

Umbilical hernias (pronounced either um-BIL-ic-al or um-bill-EYE-kall – both pronunciations are correct) are not something to worry about. They very rarely cause any trouble whatsoever, and they do not normally cause the child any pain at all. They're particularly common in:

- children of West Indian or African ancestry;
- premature babies;
- youngsters with Down's syndrome.

But they affect all ethnic and social groups. The important point to realize is that, generally speaking, they are a minor ailment.

Treatment

The great thing about navel hernias is that most of them get better on their own. In the majority of cases, the gap in the child's abdominal wall simply closes up, as his belly muscles get stronger. So the doctors will need to keep an eye on your child's umbilical hernia. But there's quite a good chance that they won't have to operate.

Note that the bulge may actually get a little bigger during the first four months or so of life. However, after that it should start to get smaller. Bear in mind, though, that it won't cure itself overnight. Very often, it takes up to three years.

You may find that older relatives or friends want you to try the traditional 'treatment' of strapping a coin across the child's belly-button. People often say confidently that this cured their Uncle Fred in 1962; they don't realize that he would have got better anyway. So coins won't do anything – except perhaps to irritate or chafe the baby.

Surgery

If the hernia doesn't seem to be disappearing, then you should take your GP's advice on whether it is worth going to see a surgeon about it. I would strongly recommend that you ask for a paediatric surgeon (if one is available in your part of the world), rather than a general surgeon.

The decision as to whether surgery should be performed is one that you should reach in conjunction with the paediatric surgeon. In general, if a navel hernia is still sticking out prominently at the age of three, then an operation is probably a good idea. One reason for this is that if your child's rupture isn't cleared up soon, then other children are going to notice it and probably make rude remarks.

The operation itself is very straightforward. It is done under a general anaesthetic, and your child will probably have to stay in hospital for a couple of days or so.

The surgeon makes a small incision in the region of the navel, pushes the hernia back inside, stitches the tummy muscles together – and then closes up the skin.

In the past, surgeons have unfortunately sometimes opted to remove the child's navel altogether, in order to get a firmer repair.

But someone whose navel has been removed looks different from other people – I have known children who've had nothing but a scar where their navels should have been, and they clearly didn't like it, especially on the beach!

So have a word with your surgeon, and make sure that he has no plans to take your child's navel away.

Paraumbilical hernias

'Para' means 'alongside', and a paraumbilical hernia is one that occurs very near the navel – usually just above it.

In contrast to umbilical hernias, paraumbilical ones don't usually cure themselves. They therefore have to be operated on, in much the same way as an umbilical hernia.

Rarer childhood hernias

Groin and navel ruptures are very common in childhood. But there are one or two rarer types of hernia which are sometimes found in small boys and girls.

Bochdalek's hernia

Bochdalek's hernia occurs in about one in every 5,000 babies. It's a congenital problem, which often has to be dealt with surgically within a few hours of birth. It's caused by a gap in the diaphragm – the sheet of muscle which makes a partition between the child's chest and his abdomen. The hole is at the back of the diaphragm.

Some of the child's abdominal organs bulge through this gap during pregnancy, crushing the lungs. This makes it very difficult for him to breathe when he is born.

Morgagni's hernia

Morgagni's hernia is rather similar to Bochdalek's hernia, but the gap is at the front of the diaphragm, rather than the back. Again, urgent surgical repair of the hole is needed.

11

Non-groin hernias in adults

Only a small minority of hernias occur outside the groin. If you have one of these non-groin hernias, but you haven't ploughed through the main part of this book, you should read Chapters 1 and 2 (or look at the summary in Chapter 12) to find out what hernias are, and what might cause them.

As for treatment – the best way of dealing with nearly all hernias in adults is to have an operation. Surgery usually cures the problem. In most cases of hernia, what the surgeon does is:

1 Makes an incision (cut) in the skin;
2 Pushes the bulge back through the gap from which it has emerged;
3 Stitches up the gap – and then closes the skin incision.

Nowadays, surgeons are sometimes able to cure non-groin (as well as groin) hernias by inserting a sheet of mesh (made of some material such as polypropylene) instead of darning up the hole.

And it's becoming increasingly common to treat non-groin hernias by keyhole surgery where possible. Keyhole (or laparoscopic) surgery avoids the need for large incisions in the skin – as described in Chapter 5.

In cases where a non-groin hernia *can't* be operated on, because the person isn't fit enough for surgery, then some form of belt or support is usually prescribed.

Types of non-groin hernia

What types of non-groin hernia are there? Figure 11 shows the possible sites of these. The following varieties occur:

- **Umbilical or paraumbilical hernias**. Umbilical hernias occur at the navel. Paraumbilical ones occur immediately next to the navel.
- **Incisional hernias**. These occur as a result of a weakness caused by a surgical operation. Figure 11 shows the site of one which

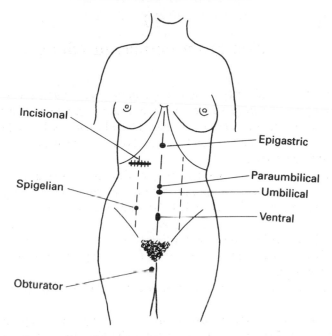

Figure 11 The sites and types of non-groin hernias.

occurred following gall-bladder surgery – though an incisional hernia can happen after all sorts of operations.

- **Ventral hernias.** These occur in a gap between the muscles of the lower abdomen, between the navel and the pubic area. But some surgeons use the word 'ventral' to mean either 'incisional' or 'epigastric'.
- **Epigastric hernias.** These are rather similar to ventral hernias, but break through in the upper part of the abdomen. Confusingly, some doctors also call these 'ventral hernias'.
- **Obturator hernias.** These are rare; they occur in a small, natural gap, located below the groin area.
- **Spigelian hernias.** These very rare hernias occur in a gap in the muscles on one side of the abdomen.

Please note that this book does not deal with the condition known as **hiatus hernia**, which is a very different type of disorder. It's the subject of another volume in the Overcoming Common Problems series (*Coping Successfully with a Hiatus Hernia*).

We'll now have a look at each type of non-groin hernia in more detail.

Umbilical and paraumbilical hernias

Childhood umbilical hernias – which are quite different from adult ones, and which often cure themselves – are dealt with separately in Chapter 10.

The navel (umbilicus) is a potentially weak spot in the front wall of the belly. Therefore, it's not surprising that adults sometimes get a rupture in this area. In fact, most such ruptures occur either just above or just below the navel. If your hernia happens to be a centimetre or two above or below your navel, your surgeon may refer to it as a paraumbilical hernia. ('Para' is just the Greek for 'alongside'.)

To all intents and purposes, we can regard umbilical and paraumbilical ruptures in adults as being the same thing: they occur in the same groups of people, and are treated in exactly the same way. During the rest of this chapter, we'll call them all 'umbilical'.

Umbilical hernias affect mainly the over-40s. They're common in women – and especially in those who have had several children. Overweight people are particularly likely to get them, as are those whose abdominal muscles have become slack.

The first thing you notice is a lump, at or very near your navel. It's usually painless – if there is any pain, you must see your doctor *immediately*. The swelling is soft, and can be pushed back inside the tummy. There's often a slight gurgly feeling on your finger-tips when you do this.

If you find such a lump, you should make an appointment to see your doctor within a week or so. She will examine you, and make sure that the swelling is indeed due to an umbilical hernia. There are one or two other conditions which cause a swelling at the navel – but in these cases, the lump is usually quite hard.

Your GP will assess whether or not you need an operation. In the vast majority of cases, you will – though sometimes, if an umbilical hernia is very tiny, it may be kept under observation for a while.

However, your doctor will almost certainly want you to go and see a surgeon fairly soon. The reason for this is that umbilical hernias in adults carry a distinct risk of strangulation. This is a very serious complication, in which the blood supply to the swelling gets cut off; it can rapidly lead to gangrene. (See Chapter 4 for more details on strangulation.)

The chief symptom of strangulation is pain. So if you've been diagnosed as having an umbilical hernia, and if you develop pain in it, this is potentially a medical emergency. Ring your doctor for advice.

Surgery for umbilical hernias

An umbilical hernia is (fortunately) easily cured – by an operation known as the Mayo repair or sometimes as the double-breasted repair. The surgeon makes a small incision across your navel, returns the contents of the bulge to their proper place inside your tummy, and then repairs the gap by overlapping two layers of your muscles and stitching them together (hence the term double-breasted). The Mayo operation – which is named after a great American surgeon, rather than the Irish county – is almost invariably done under general anaesthetic.

Your recovery time will depend on all sorts of factors – like how fit you are, and how big the hernia is. But you're unlikely to be ready to return to work within a month.

However, the long-term results of the Mayo operation are very good indeed – especially if you avoid obesity and keep your tummy muscles in good condition by taking a reasonable amount of exercise. The recurrence rate (the risk of the hernia coming back) is said to be about three per cent per year.

Recently, some surgeons have taken to repairing umbilical hernias by keyhole (laparoscopic) surgery, or by the mesh method – in which a small sheet of synthetic, net-like material is used to repair the hole. The long-term results of these newer methods aren't yet known.

Alternatives to surgery for umbilical hernias

If – and only if – a person is medically unfit for surgery, an attempt may be made to control her umbilical hernia with an abdominal support.

This is a sort of belt, rather like a corset, which is meant to put pressure on the navel – so keeping the bulge inside the abdomen. It *must* be fitted by a skilled orthotist (a specially trained technician who works in the Surgical Appliance department of a hospital).

In the unlikely event that your umbilical henia is treated with a support of this type, you must be on the look-out for pain in the region of the rupture. If it occurs, ring your doctor immediately.

Incisional hernias

Incisional hernias bulge through the site of an operation, emerging where the surgeon made his incision – and causing a lump under the skin.

They're commoner than you might think: a medical journal recently estimated that as many as one in 10 of all patients who undergo abdominal surgery may eventually develop an incisional hernia. I myself think that this assessment is on the high side; nevertheless, an incisional hernia is a possible complication of almost any kind of operation on the abdomen. (They can occasionally occur in other parts of the body too.)

Most people are very surprised to be told that abdominal surgery may be followed by a hernia. But the fact is that cutting into the abdominal wall automatically creates a potential weakness. Therefore, it's possible that some years after the operation – and occasionally much sooner – a bulge will appear at the incision site.

Operations which may be followed by the development of an incisional hernia include:

- gall-bladder removal;
- ulcer surgery;
- bowel cancer operations;
- caesarian section;
- gynaecological operations which involve cutting through the skin of the abdomen;
- appendix removal (rarely).

Fortunately, keyhole (laparoscopic) surgery is hardly ever followed by the development of an incisional hernia – mainly because the incisions in this type of procedure are so tiny.

You may well feel astonished at the idea that an incision sewn up by a surgeon could, in effect, give way, resulting in a hernia. You may well wonder whether you could sue the surgeon or the hospital if this has happened to you. Indeed, in America people who developed incisional hernias have tried to sue their surgeons. But in the UK and Ireland, it would be quite difficult for such an action to succeed in court. You would have to prove that the surgeon had been incompetent in his stitching – and that would be very hard indeed.

Furthermore, among the various causes of incisional hernia are certain factors over which the surgeon has no control – for example:

- obesity of the patient;
- coughing – often linked to smoking;
- injudicious lifting;
- poor abdominal muscles, due to lack of exercise.

Other factors which may increase the risk of an incisional hernia include diabetes, poor nutrition, treatment with steroid drugs and – very importantly – infection of the wound immediately after the operation.

Symptoms

The classic symptom of an incisional hernia is a bulge occurring in the operation scar. Depending on the extent of the original operation, the bulge may be very big. Thus, if you have a 15-centimetre (6-inch) scar down your abdomen, it's possible that you'll develop a bulge 15 centimetres long.

The swelling is soft, and it bulges out when you cough. It usually becomes more prominent if you lift your head up off your pillow. There may be discomfort, but actual pain is unusual.

Fortunately incisional hernias are only rarely subject to strangulation (so common in many other types of rupture), in which the blood supply to the swelling gets cut off. None the less, it is usually a good idea to consider having an operation to correct the incisional hernia – especially if, as is quite often the case, you have been left with a really unsightly bulge in your tummy.

Surgery for incisional hernias

There are so many different kinds of incisional hernia that it's impossible to go into detail about the possibilities of curative surgery. However, there are basically three possibilities:

1 If the hernia is quite small, and your abdominal muscles are good, then a surgeon may be able to do a fairly minor operation, in which she just removes the sac (the pouch containing the bulge), and then sews up your abdominal wall in layers.

2 If the hernia is large, it may be possible for the surgeon to do a more extensive repair of the Mayo type (described above, under umbilical hernias), in which the muscles of your abdomen are stitched together in an overlapping fashion, like the layers of a double-breasted coat.

3 If you have a very large hernia, and it would really not be possible to bring the layers of muscle together, then the surgeon may be able to repair it by inserting a sheet of synthetic mesh to fill up the gap.

You must decide what is best for you, in discussion with your GP and your surgeon. It is worth bearing in mind that the recurrence rate following repair of an incisional hernia is quite high.

If you don't have surgery to repair your incisional hernia (for instance, if you have a bad chest and are not really fit for operation), then the surgeon will probably recommend some form of abdominal support or corset. This needs to be specially fitted for you by the orthotist at the hospital's Surgical Appliance department. He may have to make an individual one for you from scratch, depending on the size and shape of your hernia.

Ventral hernias

The word 'ventral' just means 'to do with the belly'. This type of hernia causes a lump which emerges between the navel and the pubic hair – pushing out from between the two muscles which lie at the front of the abdomen.

Ventral hernias tend to occur in older people, in those who have suffered muscle wasting as a result of some serious illness, and in women who have had several children – with resultant damage to their lower abdominal muscles.

In many cases, no treatment is needed, especially if the person is not bothered by the lump. A specially prescribed abdominal support may be helpful.

Epigastric hernias

Epigastric hernias (like ventral hernias) also occur on the mid-line of the belly – but well above the navel. Sometimes they are multiple – so the patient has a line of little bumps running upwards from his navel.

For some reason, epigastric hernias are most common in younger men. The symptom they produce is a lump (or lumps). Sometimes the person also complains of pain in the upper part of the tummy – and this can actually be mistaken for indigestion.

Fortunately, many cases of epigastric hernia don't need any treatment – especially if the person is quite happy to have an unobtrusive lump located just below the tip of his breastbone. But if you want this small hernia cured, then these days it is very easy to have simple day-case surgery to repair it. Some surgeons are willing to do it by keyhole (laparoscopic) surgery, so that you are left with a very small scar and make a quick recovery.

Obturator hernias

An obturator hernia is an uncommon form of rupture. It's most often seen in elderly women.

The hernia finds its way through a tiny natural gap located below the groin and at the top of the thigh. The patient may notice a swelling, but there is a high chance she will simply complain of pain on the inside of the thigh, because the bulge is pressing on a nerve.

Obturator hernias often develop the complication known as strangulation, so they should be operated on wherever possible.

Spigelian hernias

Spigelian hernias (pronounced spy-GEE-lee-ann) are rare. They are ruptures which find a gap between the muscles of the lower part of the belly.

If you have this type of hernia, you'll develop a tender lump, located a few centimetres to one side of the mid-line of your belly, somewhere between your navel and the top of your thigh.

The cure is an operation to push the hernia back inside, and to repair the gap between the muscles.

12
Summing up

We shall finish this book by summarizing a few of the really important facts about hernias (ruptures):

- A hernia is just a bulge through a gap.
- Nearly all hernias need curing – by means of surgery (the chief exception being navel hernias in young children).
- If a hernia becomes painful, this is probably a medical emergency – get to a doctor or hospital as quickly as possible.
- The vast majority of hernias occur in the groin.
- Groin hernias aren't caused by sex – and in most cases, they will have no significant effect on the patient's sex life.
- Most groin hernias are linked to an inborn weakness in the wall of the belly.
- Other factors which can increase the risk of all kinds of hernia include fatness, heavy lifting, repeated coughing, and letting the abdominal muscles get slack and out of condition.
- Unfortunately, surgery may sometimes be followed by recurrence of the hernia.
- Recurrence is more likely if you let yourself get overweight and unfit.
- These days, you can often have some choice in what kind of hernia surgery you have – though it's easier to exercise choice if you carry medical insurance, or can afford to go privately.
- There's much to be said for the traditional operation for groin hernias – because the long-term results are well known.
- The disadvantages of traditional-style operations are that recovery is slow, and there is a moderate amount of pain.
- The newer operations, like the open mesh procedure and keyhole (laparoscopic) surgery, give you a much quicker recovery time – generally with less pain.
- The long-term results of the newer operations (and particularly the risks of recurrence) won't be known for some years.
- The new operations do offer you the advantages of day-case surgery.
- If you're considering day-case surgery, make sure that it really *is*

the right thing for you! As I was completing this book, the Consumers' Association published a survey which showed that a small but important group of surgical patients (about one in 10) wished they *hadn't* had day-case procedures, and would have preferred to be allowed a longer stay in hospital. Regrettably, most of them had been given no choice in the matter.

So you now have all the relevant facts about that common condition called hernia. What you do about those facts is (at least, to some extent) up to you. Good luck.

Useful addresses

Here are some addresses and phone numbers from which you could obtain further information. Please note that some of the names below are those of commercial firms which cannot reasonably be expected to give totally impartial advice about choice of clinic or method! I myself cannot make recommendations about particular surgeons or clinics.

Royal College of Surgeons of England
35/43 Lincoln's Inn Fields
London WC2A 3PN
Published a helpful and reassuring little booklet called *Hernia Repair Operation.*

Clarkson, Wright & Jakes, Solicitors
Valiant House
Knoll Rise
Orpington
Kent BR6 0PG
Legal firm with a special interest in medical cases.

The British Hernia Centre
87 Watford Way
Hendon Central
London NW4 4RS
Private hernia clinic, currently specializing in open mesh repair.

The London Hernia Centre
9 Hilltop Road
London NW6 2QA
Private hernia clinic, currently specializing in open mesh repair.

Hernia Awareness Line
0171 600 7374
Advice line which aims to tell you where the nearest surgeon doing the open mesh operation is to be found (UK only).

Surgical Advisory Service
0171 637 3110
Advice line, staffed by State Registered Nurses who aim to direct patients to the nearest appropriately qualified private surgeon (UK only).

Surgicare Ltd
Parkway House
Palatine Road
Northenden
Manchester M22 4DB
Headquarters of a small chain of private hernia clinics, specializing in the newer methods.

Index

Index